"Romantic partners of adults with ADHD need good information—they *really* need it. Fortunately, Tschudi's new book, *Loving Someone with Attention Deficit Disorder*, is loaded with good information. Not only is she herself the romantic partner of someone with ADD, she is also a therapist, and that clinical wisdom shines through. If you are the romantic partner of someone with ADD, you owe it to yourself to read this book."

> —Ari Tuckman, PsyD, MBA, author of *Understand Your Brain, Get More Done; More Attention, Less Deficit*; and *Integrative Treatment for Adult ADHD*

"*Loving Someone with Attention Deficit Disorder* takes the reader through the journey of recognizing and dealing with the havoc created by ADD. This book can benefit both the non-ADD individual as well as the partner with ADD. It is illustrative of the difficulties that I find in my patient population and can provide a source of knowledge, facts, and practical tools for rebuilding and enhancing a couple's relationship. I also highly recommend it for clinicians working in the field of mental health."

> —Ed S. Jesalva, MD, experienced psychiatrist and consultant

"Susan Tschudi has written a helpful book from the perspective of a non-ADD spouse. *Loving Someone with ADD* not only provides facts and refutes myths about ADD, but also gives hope to spouses and partners. She emphasizes important topics such as addiction, conflict resolution, and self-care. I recommend this book to couples in relationships wherein either one or both of the partners are affected by ADD."

> —Stephanie Moulton Sarkis, PhD, author of *10 Simple Solutions to Adult ADD, Making the Grade with ADD, ADD and Your Money*, and *Adult ADD: A Guide for the Newly Diagnosed*

"*Loving Someone with Attention Deficit Disorder* is a wonderful and needed tool for couples. First, Tschudi expands our understanding of the impact of ADHD on individuals and relationships. She then offers practical and specific coping strategies to empower couples with the skills needed to manage the challenges of ADHD together."

> —Dennis Lowe, PhD, professor of psychology at Pepperdine University and Emily Scott-Lowe, PhD, director of social work at Pepperdine University

"ADD and ADHD have damaged many relationships. Partners of people with this complicated issue sometimes take it personally or don't understand that their mate may not be in control of his or her own thought processes. Tschudi's book will help couples make sense of this misunderstood dilemma and assist them in making healthy choices about their own relationships."

> —Barton Goldsmith, PhD, author of *Emotional Fitness for Couples*

"This book will be immensely helpful if you are married to someone with ADHD. It will help you find and keep your balance. It will help you understand your partner and not act like a frustrated parent. Tschudi has written a wise, practical, and compassionate book."

> —William Doherty, PhD, professor of family social science at the University of Minnesota and author of *Take Back Your Marriage*

loving
someone
with
attention
deficit
disorder

A Practical Guide to Understanding Your
Partner, Improving Communication &
Strengthening Your Relationship

SUSAN TSCHUDI, MA

New Harbinger Publications, Inc.

Publisher's Note

Distributed in Canada by Raincoast Books

Copyright © 2012 by Susan Tschudi
     New Harbinger Publications, Inc.
     5674 Shattuck Avenue
     Oakland, CA 94609
     www.newharbinger.com

Cover design by Amy Shoup
Text design by Tracy Marie Carlson
Acquired by Jess O'Brien
Edited by Nelda Street

Library of Congress Cataloging-in-Publication Data on file with publisher

Printed in the United States of America

14 13 12

10 9 8 7 6 5 4 3 2 1

First printing

Dedicated to C. T., my favorite person with ADHD.

Contents

PART 3
Strengthening Your Relationship

Acknowledgments

I would like to thank my husband, Craig, and my kids, Jordan, Randy, Kendall, and Tyler, for all of their encouragement, support, and understanding.

Special appreciation goes to the kind people at New Harbinger Publications, who gave me the opportunity to share this information.

This book could not have been written without all of the non-ADHD partners who have honestly and courageously shared their heartaches and triumphs with me over the years. Thank you.

Introduction

In my counseling practice as a licensed marriage and family therapist, I work with couples who are trying to restore broken aspects of their relationships. While not all of the couples have attention deficit disorder (ADHD) as an issue in their relationships, a surprising number of them do. Sometimes they already know it, and other times I pick up on it and assist the couple through the diagnostic process. I have discovered that, while it is important to help the partner with ADHD to manage symptoms, it is equally important to address the frustrations and problems that the non-ADHD partner experiences; in fact, sometimes the non-ADHD partner needs counseling more than the ADHD partner does. There's no doubt that it can be difficult to be in a relationship with someone who has ADHD.

Although it is not unusual for two people with ADHD to find each other and establish a relationship, the vast majority of people with ADHD end up with a partner who does not have the disorder. I assume that you are reading this book because you are the partner who doesn't have ADHD. You probably do not struggle with distractibility, impulsiveness, inattention, or restlessness to the degree that it impairs your daily functioning, but your partner probably does. You may be well versed in the particulars involved with ADHD, or you may not know very much at all about it. Your partner may have received a formal diagnosis, or you may only suspect that ADHD is part of the problem. Regardless of where you and your partner are in the process of understanding ADHD, I trust that this book will be helpful to you in your relational journey.

I Know What You Are Going Through

On a personal level, I have come to know and understand ADHD well, but this knowledge came about by accident. When I was in graduate school, the only discussion of ADHD occurred in a class that focused on evaluating and conducting therapy with children and adolescents. I spent the required amount of time learning the symptoms and the criteria for diagnosis, but since I knew that child therapy was not going to be my professional focus, I mentally filed the information away and considered it somewhat irrelevant as a diagnostic issue for adults.

After completing my education, I began my clinical training in earnest, and during one of my first field placements in Los Angeles, I found myself counseling a very creative population. Most of my clients wanted to work, or did indeed work, within the entertainment industry as actors, musicians, directors, producers, lighting experts, set designers, and so on. Although I was unaware of it at the time, many people with ADHD are very creative, and I began to discover that many of my intensely creative clients were exhibiting some of the same symptoms of ADHD that I had studied in my graduate-school class about children and adolescents. Wrapped up and firmly entrenched in many of my clients' challenges and failures—including past academic pursuits, work-related endeavors, and especially interpersonal relationships—were many of the symptoms attached to ADHD. So I searched for as much information as possible on adult ADHD, and attended whatever seminars and workshops on the subject that were available at the time to help me understand and work with this population.

As I began to better understand the disorder and how it can affect an adult, I discussed my findings with my husband at home, usually over dinner. Time and time again, he made the comment, "That sounds like me!" and I had to agree. I don't remember the specific time or place, but at one given moment, we looked at each other and had a mutual "aha" experience. That's when the lightbulb went on for both of us. Consequently, my husband was evaluated, and the results supported our suspicions: he tested at an appreciable level for the inattentive type of ADHD. He has since found that taking medication has lessened the symptoms and helped him significantly.

Even though medication has helped my husband, there are still times when the frustration of dealing with his long-standing symptoms of distractibility, impulsivity, restlessness, and overall inattention just plain gets to me, and I become aggravated, discouraged, and angry. I have become frustrated over the years with the lack of attention paid to the non-ADHD partner and the problems this person experiences while living day to day with a partner who has ADHD.

The purpose of this book is to share helpful information I have learned about ADHD in my own life and through my clinical practice (names have been changed and situations modified to protect confidentiality). Just as I struggle to maintain healthy parameters in my personal life, I will encourage you and help you learn to do the same. It can be challenging, but in the end, it's worth all of the effort.

What to Expect

As the non-ADHD partner, if you lack knowledge about ADHD, you may be unaware of the far-reaching and sometimes detrimental impact this disorder has on relationships. You may feel discouraged and helpless to effect any change. In both my personal and professional lives, I am dedicated to supporting and helping partners to sustain healthy relationships. Therefore, each part of this book is devoted to helping you to learn more about ADHD and to discover healthier, more productive ways to survive the ups and downs of a relationship that involves ADHD.

In part 1, "Help! My Partner Has ADHD," we will examine what ADHD is and what it isn't, including a description of the different types of ADHD and a discussion about what causes this disorder.

Part 2, "Understanding Your Partner," focuses on the impact of ADHD and how the disorder affects your partner in every area of life.

Just as important, part 2 will also help you to understand how your partner's ADHD affects your life too.

Part 3, "Strengthening Your Relationship," examines solutions and skills that can help you navigate your daily life with your ADHD partner in a healthier and more constructive manner.

Let me be clear: this book is not a thirty-minute guide to understanding your ADHD partner. I wish it were that simple, but it's much more complicated than that, as you probably already know. You are invited to enter into a realistic and deeper understanding of both yourself and your ADHD partner, which takes courage, resiliency, and resolve. I look forward to sharing this journey with you.

PART 1

Help!
My Partner Has ADHD

CHAPTER 1

What ADHD Is
and What It Isn't

The problem with ADHD as a disorder is that no one can "see" it. It isn't as obvious as the debilitating symptoms of depression; depression often displays itself with sadness, lack of energy, isolation, and sleep and appetite disturbances. Also, ADHD isn't as obvious as the agitated behavior that can be associated with pure anxiety, such as excessive worry and nervousness. The basic behavioral markers generally connected to ADHD are restlessness, impulsivity, and distractibility. These characteristics play out in an adult's life as forgetfulness, difficulty sustaining attention, loss of focus, lack of follow-through, procrastination, fidgeting, impulsive speech and behavior, poor time management, moodiness, and so on (Adler 2008).

For people who don't understand ADHD, the behaviors resulting from adult ADHD can appear to be issues of character: selfishness, self-centeredness, laziness, and disrespect. Chronic and unchanging, these behaviors add to the impression of a lack of personal integrity, especially as it relates to an intimate relationship. In Karen and Bob's home, they divided up household duties equally, and it was Bob's job to take out the kitchen trash when the container was full. Karen didn't mind so much that Bob never seemed to realize that the bin was full and needed emptying, but she did begin to take offense when, after constant reminders, the trash still didn't get emptied. After a while she began to believe that Bob was exhibiting passive-aggressive behavior by ignoring her on purpose. The truth was that Bob had ADHD and tended to get distracted by something while on his way to pick up the trash can. He would get involved in whatever caught his eye, and the trash would be forgotten.

Although there are some exceptions, the perception that the behavior of a person with ADHD stems from selfishness or self-centeredness is generally untrue. If a client with ADHD is habitually late to our counseling session, I know not to assign any ulterior motive to her behavior. She is not, by nature, rude or inconsiderate; in fact, she probably had every intention to be on time. So I must remind myself that this client has ADHD and because of that—and that alone—something most likely distracted her and time got away. By examining what causes ADHD, you will realize that ADHD is not a character issue at all, but a disorder with solid neurobiological origins.

What Causes ADHD

Let's get a basic understanding of what ADHD is, according to the experts who study it. Attention deficit/hyperactivity disorder, or ADHD, is a neurobiological disorder that results in underfunctioning of specific areas of the brain. Certain neurotransmitters in the brain, called *dopamine* and *norepinephrine*, are not dispersed in an even manner, which causes the brain to underfunction. Dopamine is responsible for attention, focus, and staying on task, while norepinephrine assists with attention span, impulsivity, and distractibility (Antai-Otong 2008). The underfunctioning seems to occur primarily in the area of the brain called the *prefrontal cortex*, which is located right behind the forehead (Wadsworth and Harper 2007). The overall function of the prefrontal cortex is to assist in self-management. The brain's ability to self-manage is commonly referred to as *executive functioning*, and it is in charge of the following crucial functions:

- attention span

- judgment

- decision making

- planning

- prioritizing

- impulse control

- modulation of emotions

To put it simply, the purpose of executive functioning is to help us sort through all the different possibilities of action that crowd into the brain. Then, executive functioning helps us to make good decisions, or choose the best action or behavior according to the circumstances. Furthermore, it also helps us to set, work toward, and complete goals and objectives.

Picture an executive sitting at a big desk, and imagine all of the tasks that are necessary for getting a job done: making decisions, giving directives, managing employees, setting goals, overseeing the different departments, and directing outcomes. The ADHD symptoms of forgetfulness, difficulty with managing time, procrastination, disorganization, poor follow-through, impulsivity, and distractibility create unusual demands on executive functioning and hinder its ability to work properly, resulting in diminished ability to pay attention, make decisions, exercise judgment, and so on. The capacity to manage all of the tasks at once is compromised, and the natural flow of executive functioning is disrupted. When this part of the brain underfunctions, behaviors caused by ADHD become more evident and, in some cases, problematic.

While everyone struggles with feeling restless, being distracted, and acting impulsively from time to time, a diagnosis of ADHD is given when these symptoms create some type of impairment in a person's life. Impairment in life touches on personal, social, and occupational areas. It's not uncommon for adults with ADHD to experience issues such as chronic unemployment, job hopping, or workplace difficulties. They also might have problems with accomplishing life goals and difficulties with maintaining meaningful relationships with friends and partners (Stein 2008).

Types of Attention Deficit Disorder

ADD or ADHD? There is a common misconception that there are two separate labels for this disorder. I have heard many people say, "I have ADD; I don't have hyperactivity, so I don't have the 'H.'" To clear up any confusion, *both* terms refer to the same condition. ADHD is the accurate term for anyone who has the disorder, and that is the term that I will use throughout the book. However, the clinical diagnosis of ADHD is sub-categorized into three different subtypes, all three of which are classified as attention deficit/hyperactivity disorder. But there are different markers that create each subtype. Let's look at each in turn.

ADHD, Predominantly Hyperactive-Impulsive Type

The first type of ADHD is called *attention deficit/hyperactivity disorder, predominantly hyperactive-impulsive type*. The following are common symptoms of hyperactivity, based on the *Diagnostic and Statistical Manual of Mental Disorders*, fourth edition, text revision (*DSM-IV-TR*) (APA 2000), and the Adult ADHD Self-Report Scale (ASRS-v1.1) Symptom Checklist (Kessler et al. 2005):

- Feeling overactive or acting as if "driven by a motor" (APA 2000, 92)

- Frequently feeling restless or fidgety

- Talking too much

- Frequently fidgeting or squirming, especially using your hands or feet, when you are required to sit for long periods

- Frequently leaving your seat when you are expected to remain seated

- Frequently having trouble relaxing during free time

The following are common symptoms of impulsivity, based on the previously mentioned *DSM-IV-TR* (APA 2000) and the Adult ADHD Self-Report Scale (ASRS-v1.1) Symptom Checklist (Kessler et al. 2005):

- Frequently finishing others' sentences

- Frequently interrupting others when they are trying to focus on other activities

- Having frequent difficulty awaiting your turn

The predominantly hyperactive-impulsive type is what the general public most often recognizes as ADHD. The classic image is of a kid (usually a boy) who can't sit still in class, bothers his classmates by interrupting them, talks out of turn, makes lots of careless mistakes, and is constantly reprimanded by the teacher. Hyperactivity in adults is rare, although it does exist in some people. I remember counseling a male client with predominantly hyperactive-impulsive type ADHD who was physically incapable of sitting on my couch for the duration of an hour-long session. He would stand up, pace, and even crouch down on the floor occasionally. A few times he asked if we could conduct our therapy session outside while walking around the parking lot, because he felt so restless and wanted to move.

As a child grows into adulthood, we see fewer of the overt antics connected to hyperactivity, because the hyperactivity tends to morph into a feeling of tension or generalized restlessness (Resnick 2005). Most adults are able to moderate their hyperactivity, yet whenever I observe a person in my counseling room toe-tapping, knee-jiggling, or swinging a crossed leg, I suspect that I am observing adult hyperactivity. After I notice this behavior, I gently point it out and ask my client if he is nervous or anxious. Without exception, if the person turns out to have ADHD, he denies being anxious and adds that he was completely unaware of what he was doing. Suddenly self-conscious of the behavior, he immediately stops the bouncing or jiggling, but before too long, it starts up again. Another "diagnostic tool" in my office is one of those expandable-grid plastic toys, sitting on a table. If, during an initial session with a client, she picks it up and starts playing with it, that's also a clue that this might be another version of adult hyperactivity. I then begin taking a more detailed history that might lead to an undiscovered diagnosis of ADHD.

ADHD, Predominantly Inattentive Type

The second type of ADHD is *attention deficit/hyperactivity disorder, predominantly inattentive type*. The common symptoms of this type of ADHD, based on the *DSM-IV-TR* (APA 2000) and the Adult ADHD Self-Report Scale (ASRS-v1.1) Symptom Checklist (Kessler et al. 2005), are as follows:

- Having trouble concentrating on what people say to you, even when they are speaking directly to you

- Having problems remembering appointments or obligations

- Frequently misplacing, or having trouble finding, things at home or work

- Frequently avoiding or delaying getting started on tasks requiring lots of thought

- Having trouble setting things in order for a task requiring organization

- Having trouble paying attention when doing boring or repetitive work

- Getting easily distracted by other activities or noises

- Making careless mistakes on boring or difficult projects

- Having trouble completing the final details of a project

The person with the predominantly inattentive type of ADHD doesn't demonstrate any hyperactivity or restlessness—at least on the outside. I don't observe much toe-tapping or knee-jiggling in this type of ADHD. In fact, the person with inattentive ADHD can sit still for long periods. But he tends to struggle with what I call an "inner fidgetiness," and he experiences restlessness internally. A female client with the predominantly inattentive type of ADHD once told me that she felt as if her brain were filled with television sets, all tuned to different channels and all turned up to be as loud as possible. A casual observer would be hard put to understand this about her, because this woman appeared to be calm and collected. But her internal struggle was pure hell for her.

The inattentive type does not display very much impulsivity in word or behavior. Unlike her hyperactive-impulsive counterpart, she normally does not interrupt, speak out of turn, or butt into conversations. This person has probably never been told, "Be quiet and sit down." The inattentive type is more likely to be called a "space cadet" or may be asked, "Helloooo, is anyone in there?" because a person with this type of ADHD tends to get lost in thought and daydream a lot. To others, the person with inattentive ADHD appears to have checked out or to be mentally stuck in one place. This person is more likely to be labeled as lazy, because she tends to be rather slow-moving; she doesn't jump right into things. One might not expect the symptoms of inattentive ADHD to cause problems, especially compared to the restless and impulsive behavior associated with the hyperactive-impulsive type. But if someone is rather sluggish or slow-moving, as well as inattentive, distractible, and forgetful, this person might have chronic problems with procrastination and poor follow-through. As a result, the person with inattentive ADHD may seem to be unmotivated, unconcerned, uncaring, and nonchalant. The behavior that results from this type of ADHD is just as likely to be attributed to a lack of character.

The predominantly inattentive type of ADHD is seen most often in females and generally is not detected as early, primarily because kids with this type of ADHD don't cause any trouble in school; they are not disruptive. But when the school curriculum in the seventh or eighth grade gets more stringent, demanding more and more attention to detail, these kids tend to hit the wall academically and start to falter. Consequently, a child with inattentive ADHD who previously may have been a pretty good student starts to have academic struggles due to the fact that the schoolwork gets more tedious and boring. Remember all of those English lit novels where it takes thirty pages for someone to say hello to another person? Or how about memorizing historical facts relevant to the American Revolution? While all of this can be hard enough for most people, it feels nearly impossible for someone with the inattentive type of ADHD. When a child with undetected and undiagnosed inattentive ADHD starts to fail academically, not much consideration is given to the possibility that the cause might be ADHD. Because the symptoms of inattentive ADHD are less disruptive and don't cause any problems for others, this type tends to go under the radar. Most adults who are diagnosed with ADHD, predominantly inattentive type, are surprised that they have ADHD.

• Monica

"I have *what*?" Monica, a thirty-something-year-old woman, said in our third counseling session. She initially decided to seek counseling out of frustration with her personal life, and complained that she "couldn't get anything done." Monica's history was fairly common for someone with inattentive ADHD. She said that she had been a good student in grade school but had sort of lost her steam by the time she reached high school, and had some academic challenges that resulted in poor grades. She was well liked, had friends, and didn't have any problematic behaviors that got her into trouble. Monica enjoyed her current job, which allowed her to move at her own pace and to interact with others, but she had been let go from her previous two jobs because she couldn't keep up with production goals. Monica's home life was problematic for her; she complained that she just couldn't get a handle on things. She was disorganized, with stacks of papers everywhere and piles of things all around, plus she said she wasn't able to stay on a task for very long, especially a detailed one, no matter how hard she tried. She was behind on her taxes and had lots of late charges, because she kept forgetting to pay her bills on time.

Monica felt that she was somehow incompetent and unable to live a productive life, and she had a general sense of feeling "less than" others. She was surprised at my suggestion that she might have ADHD, because she thought that ADHD looked like "that boy, Timmy, in my fifth grade class who would never sit still, talked a lot, and got in trouble all the time." Once I explained to her what inattentive ADHD was and how it affected her life, she was very relieved. "Wow, at least I now have a name for it," was her initial response. Previously, without any understanding that her struggles were due to the neurobiological impairment ADHD causes, Monica had just tried to manage as best she could. She longed for a life that felt more personally satisfying and rewarding, but had come to think of it as an impossible goal due to her belief that there was something wrong with her. When she discovered that ADHD was at the core of her struggles, she felt renewed hope for the future.

By the time an adult gets diagnosed with inattentive ADHD, he, like Monica, has usually formed some pretty strong personal beliefs that sound something like *I'm not smart, I'm dumb, I could do so much better if only I tried harder, There must be something wrong with me*, and *I'm just bad*. Even with the new realization that ADHD has caused most of these problems, such negative beliefs can be hard to dispute, because they have existed for so long and have been reinforced along the way by parents, teachers, bosses, and even partners.

ADHD, Combined Type

We tend to think of ADHD in simple terms: a person has either the hyperactive-impulsive type or the inattentive type. Although the two types might seem to be incompatible due to the differences in behavioral symptoms, the third type, *attention deficit/hyperactivity disorder, combined type*, is a combination of the other two types. Research has shown that the combined type of ADHD is much more prevalent than one might think (Milich, Balentine, and Lynam 2001).

The person who fits the combined type of ADHD has symptoms that match the hyperactive-impulsive descriptors listed *and* symptoms that match the inattentive descriptors listed. Therefore, such a person will demonstrate both inattentive and hyperactive-impulsive behaviors. A person with ADHD, combined type, will, at times, have the "space cadet" tendency of the inattentive type but will also demonstrate the restlessness and impulsivity of the hyperactive-impulsive type.

• Leslie

Leslie, who has ADHD, combined type, would often space out in our couples counseling sessions, and it was obvious to both me and her husband that her attention had wandered off. She would get very quiet and focus on something in the room or on a part of her clothing, for example. Her frustrated husband would impatiently ask if she had heard anything he had said. Her body would literally jump, as if she had received a small electrical jolt, as her attention was pulled back into the room. She would say, "Huh? What? Oh yeah, I heard you," when it was obvious that she had been in her own world.

Leslie was definitely inattentive in our sessions, but outside of our sessions, she displayed a considerable amount of restlessness and impulsivity that was consistent with the hyperactive-impulsive type. She was constantly starting projects at home and then leaving them unfinished—all over the place. She hated housework with a passion, so she would procrastinate about doing the dishes or cleaning the bathrooms, and then find any reason at all to leave it all behind, get in her car, and go somewhere else. "Somewhere else" usually tended to be the mall, and although she wasn't extravagant, she had a big shopping problem that involved buying all kinds of unnecessary (but fun and colorful) things.

Regardless of the type of ADHD, the problematic issues surrounding the symptoms are basically the same: a general inability to pay attention for an extended period to the more mundane and ordinary things of this world, a restlessness (physical or mental or both) that makes it hard to sit still and pay attention, the tendency to get distracted by something less important and stray off target, and difficulty in thinking things through before acting on them.

The Dilemma of Diagnosing

It can be difficult to properly assess an adult with ADHD, primarily because for many years, it was thought that the disorder affected only children and that they would "outgrow" it and not be affected by it as adults. The *DSM-IV-TR* (APA 2000) provides the diagnostic criteria for ADHD that are used for all ages, but the descriptors are fundamentally related to ADHD in children. Dr. Thomas J. Spencer (2008), a psychiatrist who is an expert on ADHD, aptly describes adult ADHD as an "orphan diagnosis," because so many clinicians are not trained to recognize it in adults and tend to ignore it, trivialize the symptoms, or miss it altogether. We now know that adult ADHD is alive and well, as research shows that around 4 percent of the adult population is affected (Feifel and MacDonald 2008). Adults do suffer from ADHD, but most find ways to work around the disorder because the symptoms tend to be more varied and subtle in adults (Kessler et al. 2006).

While some ADHD behaviors are easier to notice in a school setting—sitting in a classroom all day can be very difficult for a child with ADHD—most adults with ADHD avoid anything that approximates their school experience, opting instead to work in occupations or take on endeavors that allow for some variety. The majority of my adult clients with ADHD excel in jobs where there is some sort of stimulation in the work environment. There are exceptions, but I don't know many people with ADHD who have chosen occupational pursuits like bookkeeping, engineering, or library science, for example.

As a result of the fact that ADHD was regarded for so many years as a childhood disorder, most of the questionnaires, checklists, and so on that clinicians often use to diagnose ADHD were originally created and designed for children, and little has been done to change that. The adult manifestation of ADHD seems to have been an afterthought in the mental health community. Consequently, most of the diagnostic measures may not get an accurate assessment or a good enough "read" for a proper ADHD diagnosis. As a result, the diagnosing clinician may miss the diagnosis and determine that the adult doesn't have ADHD.

If you and your partner decide that a further investigation of ADHD might be necessary, here are some things to keep in mind:

- Don't make a definitive conclusion about ADHD just by filling out a self-test questionnaire you find online or in a book. While filling out a quick and easy checklist may be useful for pointing you in the right direction, it is just a starting place.

- Find a clinician who believes that ADHD exists; understands how it can manifest in adults; will take the time to ask lots of questions about current problems; and will take a complete history.

- Accompany your partner to the evaluation and, if appropriate, to ongoing appointments. Your input as the non-ADHD partner is valuable.

What about Medication?

It's not unusual for adults who receive an ADHD diagnosis to have little, if any, understanding of the medications that are used to treat the disorder—for example, why medications are recommended, what types of medication are used, how they work, who is the best person to prescribe medication, and so on. In addition to this lack of information, there is also a great deal of misinformation among the general public, leading to negative opinions regarding using medication for ADHD. Since medication can be a crucial component of effective treatment, misinformation or lack of information can create barriers to getting appropriate help and, ultimately, to obtaining a better quality of life. Therefore, it is important to have a general understanding of medication for ADHD.

WHY TAKE MEDICATION?

Medication has proven to be an effective component of the treatment of ADHD (Dodson 2005). Medication can assist with the ability to pay attention, stay on task, and refrain from acting out impulsively. In my clinical practice, I have noticed that when a client takes the proper medication at the appropriate dose, she is better equipped to actively participate in her relationship with her partner: she can pay attention, respond appropriately, assume responsibilities, and follow through with greater ease. My client Karen, mentioned earlier, reported that after her husband, Bob, began taking medication for his ADHD, she noticed that he consistently remembered to take out the trash without any reminders (nagging) from her, and she stated that she felt better about their relationship overall. Her husband was perplexed; he didn't understand how taking out the trash could have such a strong impact, but I explained to him that his showing consistency in small areas helped relieve his wife of feeling bothered, which enabled her to concentrate on more positive aspects of their relationship.

TYPES OF MEDICATION

The following are types of medication commonly prescribed for ADHD symptoms.

Stimulants. The most common is stimulant medication (Feifel and MacDonald 2008). Stimulants are quick and predictable, with few side effects (Antai-Otong 2008). They are the first-line treatment for adults with ADHD, which means that a stimulant is usually the first medication considered because stimulants have been found to be effective at reducing the core symptoms of ADHD by targeting the underfunctioning of certain neurotransmitters in the brain.

The trade names for the most common stimulant medications marketed are Ritalin (methylphenidate hydrochloride) and Adderall (dextroamphetamine and amphetamine). While both drugs target the neurotransmitters in the brain, each has its own unique delivery system. As a result, a person may have better results with one or the other. I have had some clients who reported no reduction in symptoms when taking one stimulant but, after switching to another, experienced a noticeable and significant difference.

Because stimulant medications are fast acting, results are usually noticed within a relatively short time. If the medication is working effectively, the person should feel more focused, generally more productive at everyday tasks, and more engaged in what's going on in the immediate environment. If the medication is not working because it is the wrong medication or the dose isn't high enough to be effective, the person won't feel different or act any differently. How long a medication lasts during the course of a day depends on the type of medication; currently the extended-release versions of both Ritalin and Adderall are more popular than regular forms, because the positive effect of the medication is experienced for a longer time.

Side effects tend to be slight and transitory. Most common complaints center on loss of appetite (however, few adults really complain about loss of appetite!) and sleep disturbance. Some people report having headaches and feeling jittery and irritable. With some fine-tuning—for instance, taking the medication earlier in the day or lowering the dosage—these side effects go away.

Other medications. Several medications other than stimulants are used to treat adult ADHD, but they have been found to be less effective at reducing ADHD symptoms and can have more serious or bothersome side effects. These drugs, such as Wellbutrin (bupropion), Cylert (pemoline), and Strattera (atomoxetine) are considered second-line treatments for ADHD and are usually prescribed for adults who may have situations that preclude stimulant use, such as active drug histories, tic disorders, or certain medical conditions (Dodson 2005).

WHERE TO GET HELP

Many types of qualified health care professionals are available to help your ADHD partner manage ADHD symptoms. Although previously only medical doctors were allowed to prescribe medications, now physician assistants and nurse practitioners are authorized to do so. In some states, after completing additional training and passing an examination, clinical psychologists may now prescribe psychiatric medications on a limited basis. Regardless of the type of health care practitioner your partner works with, it is best to find one who specializes in medications that treat mental conditions, has knowledge of ADHD, and is current on the latest research and treatment. You can check the websites of national ADHD organizations, such as Children and Adults with Attention Deficit/Hyperactivity Disorder (chadd.org) or Attention Deficit Disorder Association (www.add.org), to find a referral, or ask an ADHD therapist in your area for a recommendation. Prior to making an appointment, call the office and verify that the health care professional treats adult ADHD. If not, ask for a referral within your community. It may take some effort initially, but purposeful investigation in the beginning can make medical treatment more successful in the long run.

THE BOTTOM LINE ABOUT MEDICATION

While it's not the only component in the treatment of ADHD, taking the right medication at the right dosage, at the right time, can make a huge difference in the quality of your partner's life and, consequently, the quality of your relational life. If your partner is opposed to the idea, don't get angry or discouraged and give up. Continue to educate yourself about the subject and bring it up from time to time—in a respectful and appropriate manner. Although it may take some time, raising your partner's awareness of the benefits of medication can eventually pay off.

What Doesn't Cause ADHD

Consistent scientific-research findings over many years indicate a strong neurobiological origin for ADHD (Wadsworth and Harper 2007), yet there are still many people (including in the popular media) who would like to attribute the cause of ADHD to other things, such as television, computers, diet, or the person's environment. Recently I listened to a discussion about ADHD on a local radio program, where a caller was convinced that her son's ADHD had been caused by the installation of green chalkboards and the use of yellow chalk in his school. Television, computers, and diets can feed into ADHD behaviors such as inattention, distraction, and impulsivity, but none of these factors has been able to stand alone as the explanation for or cause of ADHD.

Television and Computers

It is never good for a small child to be left unattended in front of a television, but sitting in front of a television or computer screen does not cause ADHD. There is research that has suggested this premise (Zimmerman and Christakis 2007), but other research has suggested otherwise (Stevens and Mulsow 2006). ADHD likes to be entertained, and TV shows, video games, and web surfing deliver stimulation to the brain through color, sound, and action. People with ADHD, even adults, get mesmerized and have greater difficulty with pulling themselves away from such activities. A non-ADHD client complained that one of her greatest frustrations with her husband who had ADHD was how anything on television (even commercials) could captivate him into a zombie-like trance during which he neither saw nor heard her, or anyone or anything else. She said the whole house could be coming down around him, and he would continue to stare at the screen. Another non-ADHD client told me, "Lately we seem to fight a lot about his 'electronic input needs,' and my perception that it distracts from his quality time with his family. He will sit down to dinner and play video games with his hand-held device when I'm trying to sync up with him about the day."

Diet

Some people have the opinion that a bad diet is the cause of ADHD. But a bad diet is better explained as resulting from ADHD, not causing it. People with ADHD can be food addicts due to their lack of impulse control. Fast food is just that: quick and immediate! But I have noticed a dynamic that could possibly offer another explanation. Many ADHD clients I counsel have poor diets and are drawn to sugary foods, especially those with chocolate as an ingredient, and to foods with little or no nutritional value, such as pizza, french fries, onion rings, sauces, and breads. Many of my clients tell me that after eating sugar, chocolate, or empty carbs, they feel that they can concentrate better on whatever task is at hand—at least for a while. These types of foods can help to increase arousal in the brain, resulting in improved ability to stay focused, but this ability to concentrate is short lived (Richardson 1997). People with undiagnosed and untreated ADHD are drawn to anything that they feel can help with focus and attention. I keep a candy dish in my office, and most of my clients with ADHD are often very tempted by the little pieces of chocolate.

A discussion of ADHD and food would be incomplete without some mention of specific concerns regarding food additives as the possible cause of ADHD. Studies of certain foods and additives have shown that these specific ones, at least, do not cause ADHD (Biederman and Faraone 2005). More recently, a panel convened by the FDA concluded that there is not enough evidence to prove that artificial additives contribute to such symptoms of ADHD as hyperactivity and distractibility

(Hughes 2011). No doubt the debate will continue, because some people affected by ADHD are firmly convinced there *is* a connection to food additives.

Parenting

For many years, a disruptive child who had difficulty in school or other settings due to ADHD symptoms was thought to be the product of poor parenting. Thanks to the scientific research on ADHD over the past fifty or so years, we now know that the behaviors and problems associated with ADHD are due to a neurobiological condition that has nothing to do with parenting skills. Yet many caring, concerned, and frustrated parents have felt shamed by teachers, school administrators, doctors, and others who blamed them for a child's ADHD behavior.

An examination of the strong genetic component of ADHD might help explain why this perception can occur. It is widely accepted that ADHD is highly *heritable* (Worcester 2010), which means that if a child has ADHD, there's a pretty darned good chance that at least one of his parents has it too. In fact, many of my adult clients with ADHD came to realize that they themselves had ADHD when their children went through the diagnostic process. If a child with ADHD has a biological parent with ADHD who is also the primary caretaker, then some of the dynamics of the parent's ADHD—inattention to details, distractibility, difficulty with routines and time management, and procrastination—could appear to be poor parenting and lead to misconceptions.

• Janet and Her Son

Janet, an adult with ADHD, inattentive type, and her ten-year-old son, who also has the same type of ADHD, are getting ready for work and school. Janet is tired because she got distracted by a reality TV show last night and stayed up too late, so she overslept, as did her son, since she was the one who was responsible for getting him up and going in the morning. Both of them are quickly scurrying around, trying to eat breakfast and get dressed. Janet never seems to get around to folding laundry because she hates the chore, so she and her son are rummaging through piles of clean but wrinkled clothes to try to find something to wear. Due to distractibility, Janet forgot to pick up peanut butter the day before, so she can't make her son's lunch, and she also forgot to get money from the ATM, so she has no cash to give him to buy his lunch. She will have to drop him off, go to the bank, return to the school, park the car, and run into the office to leave him some money, making her late to her first business appointment of the day.

When they finally pile into the van and head down the street, her son realizes that he forgot his backpack, so they have to return home. He begins to cry because he will be late again and the teacher gets angry when he is tardy. Janet's son has his own struggles at school due to his ADHD behavior, but if he habitually arrives late, unprepared, and disheveled, the teacher and school staff might be even more inclined to label him in a negative manner and judge Janet's parenting skills. Janet's neighbors and friends, who observe the same dynamics, may also be quick to blame poor parenting for these types of problems.

Routines and consistency are vital for creating the critical life skills of organization and planning. So, while Janet's poor organizational skills did not cause her son's ADHD, a child who already has ADHD and whose parent, as a primary caretaker, also has ADHD might be at a disadvantage for learning everyday disciplines that help create orderliness and facilitate self-management. On the other hand, if a non-ADHD parent who is better at implementing structure into daily routines is the primary caretaker of a child who has ADHD, the child might, through observation and modeling, have a better chance of learning time management and organizational habits.

What You Need to Know about the ADHD Brain

As we have learned, ADHD is a neurobiological disorder in which the neurotransmitters dopamine and norepinephrine are not regulated properly and cause the brain to underfunction. This results in the person with ADHD having a harder time paying attention and staying focused. In an effort to achieve attention and focus, the ADHD brain intuitively and consistently searches for stimulation. When stimulation occurs and the brain is engaged, it has a better chance of being able to function. Where the brain turns for stimulation depends on personal preferences; what works for one person doesn't necessarily work for another.

It is not uncommon for a person with ADHD to seek out and use some sort of substance or engage in some sort of behavior (or possibly a combination of both) to achieve stimulation. If it is a substance, it can run the gamut from cigarettes to caffeinated beverages to illegal substances. The composition of some of these substances increases arousal in the brain, which helps with the ability to pay attention and stay focused. A behavior that is used to achieve stimulation usually has a thrill-seeking component to it: driving any kind of vehicle that can go fast or be raced, engaging in daredevil stunts, gambling, and so forth. I'll cover this subject more extensively in chapter 2.

You may feel confused and wonder why your partner with ADHD feels compelled to use substances or engage in high-risk behavior. Your non-ADHD brain is much better able to stay "on point" and endure monotony, because it operates at a more consistent level. But the ADHD brain has a much harder time doing this, because the neurotransmitters do not function properly. For the person with ADHD, finding a source that provides stimulation for the brain, either through substances or activities, helps with attention and focus. Without stimulation, the ADHD brain faces monotony or boredom, and the tolerance level for monotony or boredom in ADHD is very low. The drive to get the brain stimulated is so strong that even if the substance or activity is detrimental to health or well-being, the person with ADHD may continue anyway. It is vitally important to always remember that the ADHD brain is different from yours and that you are up against a very strong biological urge. Acknowledging the difference in brain function is key to understanding not only what is going on with your ADHD partner, but also your own reactions and feelings.

For you and your partner with ADHD, there is another piece to the situation that can present just as many problems as overt stimulation-seeking behavior: anything that does *not* provide stimulation tends to be avoided, because the ADHD brain has difficulty engaging in anything that the person perceives as nonstimulating. The tolerance level for anything that the person subjectively perceives as uninteresting, tedious, or dull is very low due to the neurobiological nature of ADHD. The ADHD brain can't tolerate being bored for long and will look for a way to avoid, evade, or escape. The process of avoiding monotony or tedious-ness is, in most cases, an innate reaction that has been given very little conscious thought. Remember that when you experience something as boring or dull, you are able to deal with it more successfully because you don't have ADHD.

This can cause problems in a relationship because, in general, what-ever the ADHD brain considers boring or dull is anything that could be described as routine or detailed. For instance, activities like taking out the trash, emptying the dishwasher, remembering to run an errand, pay-ing bills, feeding the dog, sitting through a long meal with relatives—to name a few—are often forgotten, overtly avoided, or done with a lot of obvious displeasure. Because your brain does not operate in the same way as your partner who has ADHD, you don't understand, and you might tend to feel bewildered by the behavior and perhaps offended from time to time. It's very helpful to always have a filter that views ADHD, first and foremost, as a neurobiological issue, because that will help you to avoid feeling offended, resentful, or angry toward your partner. As you continue to learn about ADHD and how it manifests in your partner's life, you will be less likely to take the ADHD behaviors as personal affronts. Throughout the book we will continue to examine how ADHD behaviors are neurologically driven, and also how you can create and set in place skills that will help you to understand and cope with some of the frustrations that arise in your relationship with your ADHD partner.

PART 2

Understanding
Your Partner

CHAPTER 2

The Physical Dimension

Living with someone who has ADHD can be fulfilling and exciting, yet also very perplexing, confusing, and, at times, complicated. Many non-ADHD partners feel that life comes at them hard and fast, with little time for any thought or reflection about what is going on in their relationships. In an effort to help you sort through some of the confusion that can occur when you love someone who has ADHD, I've applied a simple, direct premise developed by psychologist Mark Laaser (1999), who recommends sometimes breaking a larger matter down into simpler elements. Examining the complex issue of ADHD in adults within the context of four basic life dimensions—physical, emotional, personal, and relational (ibid.)—will help you understand how the far-reaching symptoms of ADHD can affect the person's life and the lives of loved ones.

All of us operate within those four basic areas, or dimensions, of life: physical, emotional, personal, and relational. Trying to live life fully in each area can provoke difficulties and profound challenges without any extra dynamics involved. But when a person exhibits ADHD symptoms, managing the ups and downs of these life dimensions can be extremely demanding for everyone involved. Without a good understanding of how ADHD can affect each life dimension, lives, relationships, and families can be greatly disrupted.

To better understand this concept, try to imagine a wagon wheel. Imagine that all of the various manifestations of ADHD symptoms—disorganization, poor time management, distractibility, forgetfulness, impulsivity, procrastination, and restlessness—form the hub of the wagon wheel. Connected to the hub are the spokes of the wheel, representing the four life dimensions: the physical, emotional, relational, and personal. Because of the connection between the hub and the spokes, ADHD symptoms show up in varying degrees in all of the four life dimensions. This part of the book examines each life dimension within the context of ADHD, and I hope it will give you a deeper understanding of your partner's struggles, which can lead to greater peace and harmony within yourself and your relationship with your partner who has ADHD.

We will begin with an examination of the physical dimension. It's important to understand that distractibility, restlessness, inattention, and impulsivity can manifest in the physical dimension of life in very noticeable and obvious ways, becoming acutely pronounced and problematic. Your partner may feel compelled to engage in some activities or behaviors that will help her, at least for a while, offset the problems of distractibility, restlessness, inattention, and impulsivity in order to feel more focused and centered. Sometimes these activities or behaviors can be adaptive and helpful for this purpose. John was familiar with how ADHD interfered with his ability to accomplish work and daily tasks. He discovered that if he spent an hour each morning doing some type of high-impact physical activity, such as running or biking, his mind felt clearer and he was more successful at getting things done during the day. But many times, a person with ADHD attempts to achieve clarity and focus using methods that are not as adaptive or healthy, and those are the focus of this chapter.

Self-Medication

In the discussion of the neurobiology of ADHD (chapter 1), we learned that the irregular distribution of certain neurotransmitters seems to be responsible for ADHD. For this reason, the brain functions at a lower level, resulting in a narrower ability to pay attention and stay focused.

The ADHD brain constantly searches for something that will stimulate it, because if the brain feels as if it is stimulated, then brain functionality, the ability to pay attention and stay focused, is raised to a normal level.

Seemingly ongoing and relentless, the issues of distractibility, restlessness, inattention, and impulsivity can create a significant amount of discomfort. A person who has ADHD wants to find a way to get rid of the discomfort and, understandably, takes hold of anything that seems to get the job done. Many people with ADHD consult their doctors and are prescribed medication for this purpose, but unfortunately, many others opt to *self-medicate* to help get rid of the troublesome symptoms of ADHD. Self-medication can run the gamut, with many methods used, some legal and others illegal, but all have the propensity to become problematic.

In her book *The Link between A.D.D. and Addiction*, Wendy Richardson (1997) describes three reasons for self-medicating: to alter how we feel and how we function, to seemingly function better, and to be intoxicated. While these reasons can be applied to everyone, people with ADHD are especially susceptible to the first two reasons. Through self-medication the ADHD brain feels quieter; better able to organize thoughts and feelings; and more alert and focused and, consequently, better able to pay attention. The comment that I hear over and over again from my clients who have ADHD is "I feel *normal* after I _____" (have an energy drink, drink a pot of coffee, smoke cigarettes, throw down a cocktail or two, puff some weed, or snort a line of cocaine); in other words, "I feel *normal* after I self-medicate." The brain feels quieter for a time, and the person with ADHD is able to think more clearly, focus on one thing at a time, and complete a task. If someone who has ADHD believes that after ingesting a substance, she is able to function more efficiently, then there is less motivation to give up the substance she is using, whether it be coffee, cigarettes, alcohol, marijuana, cocaine, or anything else. The feeling of being able to perform at optimal levels is quite seductive, so it's no wonder that people with ADHD have such a high rate of substance abuse (Smith, Molina, and Pelham 2002). As with many other people, those who have ADHD also self-medicate to cope with emotional problems, but it is possible that initially, at least, the use of substances is for the purpose of offsetting the problems caused by ADHD: distractibility, restlessness, inattention, and impulsivity.

All of this is can be confusing for people who don't have ADHD, those whose brains don't function in the same way. Nancy, who was married to a man with ADHD, could never understand how her partner could drink a martini in the evening and be able to continue working for an hour or two to finish up paperwork for his job. Non-ADHD people tend to use substances to chill out, relax, settle down, or numb out. But it doesn't work the same way for people with ADHD. Their desire is to access something that will help to stimulate the parts of the brain that help them to pay attention and control their impulses. For Nancy's husband, an ounce or two of alcohol helped.

Using Substances to Self-Medicate

The methods of self-medication are on a continuum: some are not overtly dangerous, while others have the potential to greatly affect the life of the person with ADHD as well as the lives of loved ones. But anything that is used to self-medicate has the potential to be used for the wrong reasons, overused, and abused. Nicotine and caffeine, both legal substances, seem to be favorites within the ADHD population.

Tracy, a young professional woman, entered therapy for the express purpose of quitting smoking. She absolutely hated her smoking habit, and so did her husband. After we discussed the possibility that she had ADHD, she noticed that as she prepared for work in the morning, she would first shower and then walk to her closet to pick out her clothes for the day. Inevitably, she recounted, it would take her at least ten to fifteen minutes to decide what to wear. But when she lit up a cigarette right out of the shower and took a couple of puffs, she discovered that she was able to make wardrobe decisions within a few minutes. The nicotine in the cigarette worked on the neurotransmitters in her brain to create enough stimulation to allow her to focus on the task at hand. Tracy had tried just about everything under the sun to quit smoking. She and her husband were greatly relieved to discover that her addiction to cigarettes had a rational explanation. And it became much easier for her to conquer her habit when she had the proper perspective.

Another young woman, who had inattentive ADHD, stated that she could have a "serious" phone conversation with a girlfriend only after lighting up a cigarette. Otherwise she had trouble paying attention. When she realized that she was depending on the cigarettes to help her focus because of her ADHD, she became determined to find healthier ways to manage her inattention.

Robert, who had ADHD, complained that he needed gallons of coffee to be able to function, specifically to pay attention and stay on task during the day. I thought that he was exaggerating, but he reached into his backpack and pulled out a huge thermos and said that he drank four of them during the day to stay focused and on point. He was experiencing some health problems that he thought could be connected to his coffee habit, and wanted to find some way to break his dependency.

One male ADHD client proudly proclaimed that he never used alcohol or any illegal drugs, had never smoked, and didn't even drink coffee. But further inspection revealed that he regularly took an over-the-counter headache remedy (even when he didn't have a headache) that is known to have a substantial amount of caffeine as an ingredient. He washed his pill down with a 12-ounce can of a popular energy drink loaded with 32 milligrams of caffeine. When he realized how much caffeine he was ingesting every day, he was very surprised.

Even certain foods provide some relief from the frustration of inattention and restlessness that accompanies ADHD, as I have discovered. Jessica was about one hundred pounds overweight when she sought out my therapy services. After doing a complete history, I began to suspect that she might struggle with ADHD, but she had none of the regular addictions that I usually observe in ADHD clients: she had never even considered drugs, hated alcohol, never smoked, and didn't drink coffee or even caffeinated soft drinks. It was obvious that she had a food addiction, so I began to ask what her favorite foods were, and she responded that she craved sugar all of the time. Compulsively she would eat candy, pastries, or anything that was sweet and sugary. She also had a special fondness for anything loaded with carbohydrates that had little nutritional value, especially pizza and breads with sauces and gravies. Generally someone with an eating disorder might eat for comfort or for emotional reasons, but Jessica reported that her main incentive was being able to get through her day with more ease; she felt able to concentrate or stay on task better whenever she ate a lot of these particular foods. But then the sugar or empty carbs would wear off and "drop" her on her "butt" (her words), so she felt inclined to eat them again. Indeed, Jessica's brain was benefiting temporarily from the sugar and carb load, which helped her to feel calmer and more focused. After a thorough evaluation, she was found to have ADHD, inattentive type, so she sought out appropriate care, which included medication that helped improve her ability to concentrate. With a better understanding of what was driving her food addiction, she then had the courage and stamina to undergo a surgical procedure and drop the extra weight.

The overuse of substances such as caffeine and nicotine, and even certain foods, is not uncommon with ADHD, but it's also not unusual, and even quite common, for people with ADHD to use more significant substances for self-medication (Wadsworth and Harper 2007). Often, during an initial session with a client, I may suspect that ADHD is an issue, so as I take the person's history, I spend more time asking questions about past drug or substance use. I often find that normal drug "experimentation" (especially with alcohol and marijuana) that usually begins around junior-high age has turned into serious abuse or dependency in adult life. Alcohol and marijuana seem to be popular choices for a couple of reasons. First, both are easily accessible—even for a kid, unfortunately—but more important, as some of my clients report to me, there seems to be something about each substance that helps to stimulate the brain, allowing for better concentration and focus. Many of my clients have expressed that for the first time in their lives, something helped them to feel "normal"; they didn't feel as physically or mentally restless, they could start and finish something, they could sit still for a while, and they could pay attention—finally. That can be a powerful moment.

I remember a client named Anna who was a recovering alcoholic when I began treating her. With a history of failed relationships and suffering from emotional problems, she entered therapy to "work on herself." After getting to know her a little better, I began to believe that it was possible that she had ADHD. One clue was Anna's statement that she noticed that when her friends drank a bottle of wine, they would pass out on her couch, but when she used to drink a bottle of wine, she would clean her apartment, which she liked being able to do. Although she had gone on to use alcohol excessively and for other reasons, her initial attraction to this substance was that she felt "normal" when she drank and found that one benefit of feeling "normal" was that she could begin and finish tasks more easily.

One of the most compelling stories that illustrate how self-medication can be a powerful force came from a man named Calvin. He and his wife initially came to me for couples counseling. During the course of our first few sessions together, I began to detect that ADHD might be an issue for Calvin. At age thirteen, he had been offered a marijuana cigarette. He had tried it and liked it because it had made him feel what he called "normal," which meant that he seemed to be able to function better while under the influence. So he began to smoke weed almost every day before he went to school. Here's the important part: he said that in middle school, he had been a pretty good student, but when he had used marijuana daily, he had become an A student. Calvin also said that he had been a pretty good athlete, but after initiating his love affair with weed, he could "slam the ball just like Jimmy Connors." In high school he had made the varsity tennis team as a freshman. His increase in mental and physical abilities while under the influence had seemed to work well for him, although he had felt confused by observing his buddies acting stupid or stoned whenever they smoked marijuana. Although Calvin had felt sort of freakish, his newfound ability to perform really appealed to him, as you can imagine.

He continued regularly using marijuana for many years until—uh-oh!—he got married. Smoking marijuana was completely out of the question for her, almost on the same level as infidelity. To his credit, Calvin stopped—for a while—but then a demanding circumstance would arise, prompting him to sneak some weed in order to feel equipped (focused and attentive) to handle the challenge. Inevitably his wife would discover a telltale sign, like a "roach" mistakenly left in the car ashtray, and World War III would ensue. This couple was literally on the brink of divorce over his marijuana use. Calvin obtained the proper ADHD diagnosis and treatment, which included the right medication at the correct dosage, and his desire for marijuana diminished. More important, his wife was able to understand the neurobiological components of ADHD, which helped to explain his continued use, and this understanding helped her to have more compassion for Calvin.

While marijuana can create many problems and alcohol use can do great damage, many people with ADHD do not limit their substance use to alcohol and pot. Although it's less common, it is not unusual for people with ADHD to use far more dangerous and debilitating drugs for self-medication. The use of cocaine, crack, and ecstasy can lead to serious problems and may cause the non-ADHD partner to end the relationship in order to save the family. Be sure to take chronic abuse of any substance seriously and take steps to address the problem.

Using Behaviors to Self-Medicate

The physical dimension is defined by what we do—with our bodies, with our energy, and with our time. Some people use behaviors to self-medicate, to get the stimulation that allows the brain to feel focused and on task while doing the behaviors. Taking the form of hobbies or recreational pastimes, these activities can be good and healthy, providing balance in a person's life. But if the primary purpose of these activities is to provide stimulation to the brain and it results in less attention paid to work responsibilities or interpersonal relationships, then even good and healthy behaviors or activities can become problematic. Eleanor's husband, who had ADHD, loved to run, and she was glad he enjoyed a healthy activity. But she complained, "My spouse missed many family activities as our children were growing up, because he was off on four-hour trail runs in the mountains."

RECKLESSNESS

To stimulate the brain, some people with ADHD gravitate toward thrill-seeking activities that have an element of danger in them, such as motorcycling, bungee jumping, or just plain fast driving. I asked one of my young male ADHD clients what he liked to do for fun with his friends. I thought he would say hiking or playing ball, but he said he and his buddies liked to get up on Saturday mornings, get in their cars, and drive to the top of a well-known winding, rather treacherous canyon road in the community where he lived. But they didn't go there to hike or bird-watch or just enjoy nature. Their purpose in going up to the top, he said with a smile on his face, was to drive down the other side of the winding, treacherous canyon road *as fast as possible*. I asked him how his mind and body felt during the fast drive down the canyon road. He leaned back, smiled again, and said that it was the greatest sensation ever, that both his mind and body were completely focused on what was going on. But he added that his girlfriend often cried when she knew he planned to go "fun driving," as he called it, and she usually wouldn't talk to him for a couple of days afterward. Although he didn't like to upset her, he felt compelled to keep doing it because it felt so good to him.

Andrea dreaded road trips or even trips across town on the freeway with her ADHD husband. She accused him of using any driving time in the car as a mock tryout for the Indy 500 and said she had to take anti-anxiety medication every time she got in the car with him for an extended period. Many a spouse has threatened to leave the relationship because of the aggressive, dangerous driving of an ADHD partner. Indeed, people with ADHD are at a greater risk of being involved in a motor vehicle crash, drinking and driving, and traffic violations (Feifel and MacDonald 2008).

VIDEO GAMES AND THE INTERNET

One behavior that is a strong lure for the ADHD brain—because it offers such a strong delivery of stimulation—is video games, and another is Internet use. Many non-ADHD partners have complained to me about their ADHD partners' incessant fascination with video games, and they describe it as an addiction: "He sits in front of the TV or computer screen all the time. And if I didn't nag and complain, he would sit there all day long, preferring to play those stupid video games than be with me or our kids!" Video games deliver all the goods to someone with ADHD. They are colorful, loud, and fast moving, plus they create a competitive atmosphere—all components that can deliver a very quick and effective dose of stimulation to the brain. And any type of Internet activity can provide the same stimulation. One female client with ADHD sits fascinatedly surfing the Internet for hours on end. Then she suddenly realizes that it is four o'clock, dinner hasn't been started, the house is still a mess, and, even worse, the kids were supposed to be picked up at three thirty.

SEX

By the time a couple engages my services as a marriage counselor, their sex life is usually close to nonexistent. Most couples have stopped having sex because one partner is angry or hurt, or perhaps withholding sex is being used as a punishment. But I have noticed that with couples in which one partner has ADHD, there is a different sexual dynamic involved. In my clinical experience, it's not unusual for such a couple to experience some level of sexual dissatisfaction that seems to be based in boredom, which is another way of describing lack of brain stimulation. Quite often I hear these complaints: "Whenever he gets bored, he wants to have sex," "He's bored with the type of sex we have; he says he wants it more exciting," "No matter what I do, he's never satisfied," or "She says sex with me is boring; I take too long."

Can sex be used to self-medicate? You bet. Sexual stimulation generally begins as a mental process. A partner can provide easy access for the excitement and physical stimulation that occurs with sexual activity, but as some of the complaints describe, normal sexual activity sometimes isn't enough to satisfy the ADHD brain. One couple I worked with was at odds because the husband, who had ADHD, wanted to have sex every day. Despite the fact that they had a small child and an infant who didn't sleep through the night, he would get very angry when his wife wouldn't comply. And he not only wanted to have sex every day, but also complained that she wasn't willing to be inventive enough. She loved her husband but was frustrated with his demands.

The craving for brain stimulation can easily lead to viewing pornography. While a couple might use pornography to enhance their sexual relationship, pornography is usually not well received by the nonviewing partner and subsequently presents its own set of problems to a relationship by creating a world of fantasy for the viewer that can't be replicated in real life. So while it does provide an almost instantaneous dose of stimulation to the ADHD brain, pornography can have many unfavorable consequences, especially in a relationship.

LESS-OBVIOUS BEHAVIORS

So maybe your partner with ADHD doesn't jump out of airplanes or play video games all weekend. Perhaps you don't have any complaints about your sex life with your partner. There can still be subtle, less-obvious ways that a person with ADHD self-medicates by seeking out and finding something stimulating to help the brain feel less restless and agitated.

Imagine a stay-at-home mom with ADHD pondering a sink full of dirty dishes—not too exciting or stimulating, right? But wait! Suddenly she remembers that she needs to get some new sponges, so she goes to a discount store. Once she's at the store, she spends a couple of hours roaming the aisles looking at all of the bright and attractively packaged items, and impulsively buys many things other than sponges. She may even forget to buy sponges because she's been distracted by all of the other colorful things she sees. This woman's husband comes home to a dirty, messy house and several shopping bags full of new things. Depending on how long this dynamic has been going on, he might feel a great deal of frustration and even voice his frustrations in an unpleasant manner. His wife doesn't mean to make him angry, but the strong drive to find something to stimulate her brain and calm its restlessness keeps creating scenarios in which she leaves ordinary tasks behind and goes somewhere or does something more interesting and stimulating.

Another example, yet a little more puzzling, was the case of Laurie and Hugh, a couple I treated for marital problems. Hugh had ADHD, inattentive type. He didn't do anything dangerous or thrill seeking, so there were no complaints from his wife about that. In fact, he was a real homebody, or rather a real "garage body." Even though he was at home a lot, especially on weekends, he spent the vast majority of his time out in his garage, where he would tinker with his truck or work on some house project. Laurie complained that she regularly felt like a single mom because Hugh spent so little time with the family. Although he was loath to admit it, he confessed that he often felt uncomfortably restless and agitated, even around his wife and children. Hugh didn't smoke, drink, gamble, or do any of the more common self-medicating activities or behaviors usually seen in the physical dimension. But when he was able to retreat to the garage, where he could tinker with his truck and work on home projects, his brain was provided with enough stimulation to counteract the restlessness he often felt.

The biggest problem with most of the activities or behaviors that a person with ADHD uses to self-medicate is that many of them have an addictive component. You may notice that your partner's use of a substance or the repetition of a behavior may need to be increased in order to achieve the same effect in your partner. Addiction or addictive behavior causes anxiety and fear in the non-ADHD partner, because watching someone spiral out of control and refuse to come to terms with a behavior is a frightening, helpless feeling. You may suspect your partner doesn't care enough to stop the using or control the urges to smoke, drink, eat, and so on. You may think that your ADHD partner is weak willed and just doesn't try hard enough. It is absolutely essential to consider that self-medication for someone with ADHD could be, at least initially, an effort to raise brain function to a normal operating level.

Can you recognize any self-medicating activities or behaviors in your ADHD partner? Does your partner drink too much? Shop too much? Eat too much? Watch too much TV? Play too many video games? Spend too much time on the Internet? Keeping in mind some of the examples given in this chapter, make a list of all of your partner's activities or behaviors that you may perceive as bothersome or problematic. Take a look at each one and then put it through the filter of self-medication to see if your partner may be attempting to raise her level of brain activity with her behavior. Any new realizations of what may be motivating your partner can create new opportunities that will help you to work together to find solutions.

CHAPTER 3

The Personal Dimension

The spectrum of challenges caused by ADHD in the personal dimension of life is wide and varied, encompassing areas such as educational efforts, jobs and vocational interests, spiritual pursuits, and an overall sense of personal satisfaction. An examination of the personal dimension can yield an understanding of how your partner may feel about his ability to move forward in life and accomplish goals. All of the symptoms of ADHD—impulsivity, restlessness, distractibility, disorganization, procrastination, difficulty with follow-through, and issues with time management—can strongly manifest in the personal dimension.

School Performance

School experiences, even early ones, can continue to affect people with ADHD far into adulthood. Almost all of the adult clients with ADHD whom I have worked with report some sort of trouble getting through school successfully, regardless of intelligence level. Even if they did well academically, very few of them enjoyed school; in fact the majority report that they greatly disliked it, found it boring, and got tired of teachers and administrators thinking they were either stupid or lazy. When I am gathering information during an assessment for ADHD, I always ask clients to think back to grade school and try to remember what the teacher wrote in the "comments" section of their report cards. If a person has ADHD, the response—almost without exception and with very little hesitation—is "Johnny could do so much better if only he tried harder." Unfortunately, no one realized or acknowledged that Johnny was not only trying as hard as he could, but also battling the neurobiological disorder called ADHD, which affected, to some degree, his ability to successfully do the things kids are supposed to do in school: listen to the teacher, pay attention in class, remember what to do next, turn in homework, and comprehend reading assignments.

Educational struggles and difficulties in school seem to be a hallmark of ADHD (Ramsay 2002). People with ADHD, predominantly hyperactive-impulsive type, fidget and move around a lot, while people with ADHD, predominantly inattentive type, quickly begin to daydream and get lost in their own thoughts. Both types can find it hard to pay attention to the teacher, whose voice begins to sound like "Blah, blah, blah" before too long. Unless a child's hyperactive-impulsive type of ADHD limits his ability to stay in his seat during class or curb impulsive speech, most ADHD kids do pretty well in elementary school. There is a lot of "handling" of the child and a lot of internal structure in place in the lower grades. Usually there is only one teacher and one classroom, so daily routines aren't disrupted as much. There is plenty of time spent on the playground, where children are encouraged to run and play. Teachers' expectations are not as high in elementary school, and the curriculum is less stringent. At home, parents are expected to be more involved; they organize belongings that go to and from school, and regularly monitor homework. Transition to middle school can be quite difficult, especially for the child who has ADHD. Many parents are confused when, suddenly, their child is having problems at school or is in danger of failing academically.

From the ADHD child's perspective, the educational experience transforms dramatically at the middle-school level for many reasons. There are more structural changes that demand transitions—more classrooms, more teachers, and more kids in each class—adding a barrage of noisy and confusing stimuli for the brain to sort through. Each teacher has different demands and a different teaching style, creating more opportunities for a student with ADHD to become distracted. The curriculum becomes harder and more tedious. History textbooks present challenges, with the pages and pages of "boring" facts and names that all sound the same. Memorizing data for tests gets more difficult. Recess and playtime disappear, leaving fewer opportunities to burn off physical energy. In fact any physical activity is now relegated to P.E. (physical education) class, which also becomes more structured and controlled. Art and music classes are usually eliminated at this point. Anything that could have brought some stimulating enjoyment in the school setting for the student with ADHD dries up and disappears.

Now on her own, with less involvement and less monitoring from teachers and parents, the student with ADHD is more likely to forget to bring home or return to school necessary items, such as homework or assignments. Daily tracking of notebooks, textbooks, and belongings becomes more and more difficult. Teachers in middle school and high school are more critical of a student's performance and more unforgiving about missed or late schoolwork, and so are most parents. Information comes fast and furious, and because of the tendency to get distracted and miss what the teacher says, the student with ADHD can fail to notice important information that can significantly affect grades and overall school performance. This can be tremendously frustrating for the student because she knows that her poor school performance and the grades that may reflect it are not a result of any lowered intellectual capacity. Most people with ADHD are at least as smart as everyone else and entirely capable of successfully understanding the material at hand. But the challenges the student faces at school that are rooted in ADHD hold her back and make her feel trapped.

Consequently, many adults with ADHD tend to shy away from any endeavors that might have similarities to their school experience. Higher education may not even be a consideration or, for that matter, any type of profession that requires extra or ongoing training or certification (unless it involves a specific area of interest). Because of unpleasant past school experiences, your partner may impose her own restrictions that could rule out other opportunities that might become available. For the same reason she might sabotage any possible chances to advance in her profession or even, for that matter, find a profession that could bring more fulfillment. It may be upsetting for you to recognize that her potential is limited by her feelings about her earlier school experience, yet to know that her capabilities remain untapped.

Unfortunately your partner's negative school history can create long-lasting negative beliefs about his abilities that can contradict reality. Many people with ADHD emerge from their school experiences doubting their own ability to achieve and be successful. Why would your partner, who has been told for many years that he could have done so much better if only he had tried harder (when he was trying as hard as he could), feel any different about other endeavors in his life? The reality may be that your partner is intelligent and quite capable of finding success, but his negative self-talk that began a long time ago can continue to affect his thoughts, feelings, and day-to-day behaviors. I have heard many clients with ADHD tell me how something was impossible for them: "I can't do that. I'm not smart enough; why would I even try?" or "That's for smart people, not for me." You may hear your partner recite this self-defeating script over and over again. Frustrated, you may see your partner much more realistically, but he just can't see it. His vision of himself has become constricted.

Your partner's personal hopes and aspirations can also be hijacked by her lack of understanding of the limitations caused by ADHD symptoms, and this alone can set the stage for replaying the same scenario in other life endeavors in the personal dimension. But things can change once a person learns more about ADHD.

• Carl

Carl, a young man who came to me for counseling, had undiagnosed and untreated ADHD, and had been floating from one low-level job to another for several years, never feeling fulfilled or satisfied. He had not done well in school, and he felt that his teachers had given up on him. In fact, his guidance counselor had discouraged him from even considering college. His wife had recently read a magazine article about adult ADHD, which was how my client found his way to my office. After an initial diagnosis of ADHD, predominantly inattentive type, I referred him to a doctor.

With medical treatment and continued therapy, his life began to change. The dark cloud of self-doubting thoughts about his capabilities began to dissolve, and he discovered that he was not "dumb" at all but that his ADHD limited his ability to pay attention in certain settings. Relieved, he realized that most of his school troubles had been caused by ADHD rather than not trying hard enough. Carl had always had a fascination with the justice system but thought he would just have to content himself with watching television shows about courts and trials. With his newfound understanding of ADHD, he was able to seek out the help he needed, and wound up enrolling in a local junior college that had special accommodations for students with ADHD. He began the process of getting a degree and the special training that would allow him to work within the court system.

Job Difficulties

One of the biggest issues often associated with ADHD in adults is vocational challenges (Painter, Prevatt, and Welles 2008). These challenges, most often experienced as chronic job dissatisfaction, can lead a person to job-hop or to somehow get fired a lot. Some of the same problems experienced in school are also evident in job performance. For example, a person with ADHD may have a lot of trouble sitting through meetings. She may easily get bored, distracted, and fidgety. Her mind may drift away, which may be obvious (and even irritating) to the other people in the room. She may also be inattentive to work details and exhibit poor follow-through—for example, forgetting to turn in an invoice or leaving major points out of a report, which can negatively affect not only her but also her team or department. Because of impulsive language, she might have a tendency to speak before thinking, mouthing off to a boss or supervisor, or making inappropriate comments to coworkers. Disorganization in the work environment may result in a messy, cluttered workstation, where important papers are buried under a stack of unfiled memos, or perhaps important e-mails remain unopened and ignored for a long time. And time-management problems may manifest at work; for example, being late in the morning or late to important meetings, or forgetting meetings altogether. Each of these issues can cause major disruptions in a person's work environment, resulting in poor reviews, layoffs, or firings. Even though the person with ADHD may be quite talented and uniquely suited for the job in many ways, these ongoing problems get in the way of those talents being appreciated and recognized.

Someone with ADHD might settle for a job that holds little danger of being fired but may be boring and unfulfilling. In some cases he will stick with the unrewarding job because it provides a steady income for the family. William, who had ADHD, had worked his way down to a menial job. His ADHD symptoms of inattention to details, distractibility, and forgetfulness were primarily to blame for his getting either fired or laid off from previous jobs. While he was frustrated because he felt that his intelligence and abilities were significantly underused in his present job, he held on to it because it put "food on the table," as he said. William's wife, Ingrid, tried to be understanding and encouraging, but down deep she felt a little embarrassed by what he did for a living. A situation such as this, which is caused by a partner's ADHD, can disrupt relational harmony, adding another layer of frustration to the relationship.

Many non-ADHD partners, with good intentions, assume too much responsibility in the relationship and counteract their partners' employment difficulties by taking on too much work or staying in an unfulfilling job. One non-ADHD partner whom I counseled held a very important, demanding, and responsible position that paid a very good salary. She was exhausted and stressed from doing way too much: working, handling the household, and managing their two small children. Part of the reason she took on the demanding job and stayed with it was her husband's ADHD. He had a long history of many jobs that he had either left out of boredom or been fired from due to poor performance. When I counseled them, he complained about his nine-to-five job, which he hated because he felt it did not use his gifts and talents (it didn't). As a result he was always teetering on the brink of being fired or conveniently laid off. Consequently, although his wife would have loved to quit her job and search for one that was less stressful and more compatible with her children's schedules, she stayed with her stressful, unfulfilling job because she was constantly afraid that her ADHD husband would become unemployed. He was unhappy, and she was constantly edgy and anxious. Both felt that they had no control over their lives, and the stress and strain on their relationship was tremendous.

Missing the Mark

Over the years, I have counseled many people who qualify for a diagnosis of ADHD. Some are young and some old. Some are brilliant, while others are of average intelligence. Their individual stories are varied. Many have a history of educational failures, but some hold doctoral degrees. Some struggle to make a living, while others are quite successful in their chosen fields. But I have discovered over the years that all of them share an overall sense of personal dissatisfaction. Regardless of how accomplished or successful they might appear to the world, all of them, without exception, often describe a feeling that there is something important they have missed out on, that there is something just beyond their reach. This seems to be a common grievance among the adult ADHD population (Painter, Prevatt, and Welles 2008). What I hear time after time is a throwback to the old classroom criticism that becomes internalized as an adult: "I know I could do so much better if only I just tried harder or put forth more effort." This feeling is deep and profound, causing a sense of sadness and melancholy, which can greatly affect other endeavors and pursuits in the personal dimension of life.

• Emily

Emily, a woman I counseled several years ago, ran a very successful event planning business. It was a perfect fit for her and her ADHD, because it allowed her to access her creativity. In addition, each event was different from the previous one, thus providing a measure of excitement and stimulation. Being very savvy, Emily understood some of the limitations she faced because of ADHD, so she surrounded herself with assistants who were organized and detailed oriented. It was a great combination, and as a result, she had become renowned in her community as the premier event planner.

However, I began to dread any sessions with Emily that followed one of her big events. Invariably, she would show up distraught beyond reason. As we debriefed, she would discount any positive feedback she had received and instead focus on what she thought she had missed. When I tried to help her determine what it was that she thought she had missed so that she could avoid missing it the next time, she could never pinpoint the problem and usually responded, "It's just a feeling; I just know there was something else I should have done." She was so disturbed by this that she considered giving up her business altogether. Fortunately, when she began to understand that her sense of "missing the mark" was a manifestation of her ADHD, she was able to overcome her distress and frustration.

This sense of missing the mark can affect the way a person looks at life. Because ADHD can shape self-worth, often some circumstances, situations, and events aren't viewed realistically, as we saw with Emily. Throughout the years, her struggle with ADHD had conditioned her to look over her shoulder, because she believed that surely, no matter how hard she had tried, she had forgotten something important and someone was going to find out. Failing to acknowledge her success, she was convinced that she could not do a competent job, which consequently led to her inaccurate self-assessment. Emily had very little tolerance of her own shortcomings and had a tendency to hold little pity parties from time to time. Her partner was sympathetic to a point, but often displayed irritation because reality just didn't support Emily's worries. Because ADHD has such a strong impact on the personal dimension, people with the disorder are at risk of letting failures or perceived failures, rather than reality, define them.

Difficulties with Spiritual Disciplines

While often overlooked, spiritual beliefs are an important factor in the personal dimension of life and therefore deserve some discussion. Though spiritual beliefs are highly personal, a recent poll by the Pew Forum on Religion and Public Life (2010) found that most people have a belief in God or a universal spirit. Furthermore, most expressions of faith encourage followers to try to experience a higher level of spiritual satisfaction. To do this, people generally use some type of prayer or meditation and, if their particular expression of faith calls for it, the study of religious writings. I have discovered that these methods can be extremely difficult for a person with ADHD, which, at times, can cause problems in a relationship.

Prayer and meditation generally require quiet and still environments. Although there can be exceptions, this can be particularly tricky for a person with ADHD, who usually prefers to occupy his time with interesting stimuli and does not enjoy having quiet and stillness. Prayer requires concentration and focus, which can be challenging for the ADHD mind due to distractibility. Meditation necessitates clearing the mind of distractions, but it can be hard for someone with ADHD to clear his mind enough to concentrate on an important conversation with his partner, much less to meditate in total silence. By and large, religious writings are not very exciting or thrilling and may be written in outdated language. Since a person with ADHD may not be the best reader in the world, the study of religious writings may not hold his interest for long. All of these approaches—prayer, meditation, and study—have innate components that could be considered tedious and that can translate as "boring" to a person with ADHD.

So if someone with ADHD experiences difficulty in praying or meditating because she gets distracted or if she finds it difficult to study or read spiritual material because it's too dry, tedious, and boring, she may tend to steer clear of any spiritual pursuits at all. Your partner with ADHD, who may already carry a feeling of being "less than" other people in other personal pursuits, might now also feel the same way about her relationship with her higher power. The consequences of this problem can be profound and can have a significant effect on her essential beliefs about her worth and value.

If you choose to follow a spiritual path that includes attendance at a house of worship, your partner with ADHD might be unlikely to want to join in this activity, which usually requires sitting and listening to one person talk for a prolonged period. Your partner may prefer to spend time doing things that are more subjectively interesting (playing golf or watching sports on TV are two things that come to mind). This can create conflict in your relationship because you may have an expectation or desire for a shared spiritual journey, which might include attending religious services or other joint experiences with your partner. You might interpret your partner's reluctance and apathy as a lack of caring for you and your relationship.

All of your partner's struggles that materialize in the personal dimension of life can affect your life too. You can do very little to erase the negative impact of school experiences, and you can't go to work with your partner to make sure he stays on task. In most cases you are powerless to do anything and must stand by and watch while he finds his own way through his personal predicaments. The greatest contribution you can make to the relationship is to offer genuine empathic understanding. Empathy is not sympathy or feeling sorry for your partner, but is more of an effort on your part to understand his experience with sensitivity. I coach many non-ADHD clients on how to express empathy, using statements such as "This must be really hard for you" or "That's got to be really tough." Empathy communicates caring, is nonjudgmental, and can go a long way in cultivating more harmony in your relationship. If your empathy level is low, try to think of ways to be a source of encouragement to your partner, assuring him of his good qualities and affirming what you know is good about him, even if he doesn't believe you.

CHAPTER 4

The Relational Dimension

Even though your partner's ADHD-driven behaviors may not be as obvious or problematic at work, in social situations with friends, or in other settings, they can still create distress when you have to live together. Other people in your partner's life do not have the same interactions with your partner and so do not experience her ADHD in the same way that you do. At work your partner may fear being put on probation or fired, so she may be more aware of her ADHD behavior and therefore exercise more control to keep it from interfering with job performance. And if your partner is fortunate enough to work in an environment where she is given some autonomy and can access a good support staff, the ADHD-driven behaviors might cause very little trouble, if any at all. Jackie's partner was a successful entrepreneur who never had to answer to a boss or a committee and had the resources to afford an excellent assistant, so everything went very smoothly for him as CEO of his own company. But his inability to organize things at home, handle details, and be appropriately accountable to Jackie created a lot of strife between them.

An intimate, committed relationship also has different parameters than a friendship. Your ADHD partner's friends and acquaintances may love to have her around due to her spontaneity (or impulsivity). But spontaneity can be problematic at home if your partner consistently chooses to do something fun and exciting instead of holding up her end of relational responsibilities. Ronald's partner, Eileen, was hardly ever home in the evening due to spur-of-the-moment activities that she found more interesting and stimulating. His growing resentment of her, because of her choices, was affecting their relationship.

The reality is that you live with a person who may have some degree of difficulty navigating daily life due to the symptoms of ADHD. The impact of these difficulties is experienced more acutely in the relational dimension, because the fundamental nature of a committed relationship requires that two people live together in an intimate setting.

Universal Complaints

When a couple arrives for our first counseling appointment, I begin the session by asking, "What is going on in your relationship that brings you here?" I want to hear, in their own words, what they think might be causing their problems. Consequently, at least at first, I hear a lot of complaints. What I have discovered is that the complaints that tend to cluster around ADHD issues have a commonality to them that is different from complaints where ADHD is not part of the problem. There may be different variations, but they all sound the same. What's more, these common complaints seem to exist in a relationship involving a partner with ADHD regardless of any other dynamics involved: age, socioeconomic status, intelligence, culture, and so on. To illustrate how ADHD can affect the relational dimension of a partnership, I've compiled a list of some of the most common ADHD complaints that are shared with me in counseling sessions.

Inability to Remember Being Told Things

Josh, the non-ADHD partner, sat in my office with his wife and described the latest situation he had encountered with his wife's forgetting something important: "Last Friday night was my turn to have my buddies over for poker. We take turns hosting, and I had it on my calendar. That's how I *know* I had told Christy about it earlier in the week, because I've learned to make sure I tell her what's on my calendar every week. I thought she would remember, because she looked me straight in the eye when I told her and said, 'Okay, that's fine.' Usually, when she looks at me, I can count on her remembering, but I should have known—and I should have followed up." Josh was upset because Christy had forgotten about his poker game and had scheduled to have all of the carpets in the house cleaned that day. When Josh had arrived home Friday after work, he discovered that the carpets were still wet from cleaning and the furniture couldn't be put back into the rooms until the next day. "You never told me" was Christy's response. She had no memory of Josh's reminder. Josh was livid as he turned to me and said, "Yes I did! It was Monday morning before I went to work, she was reading the paper at the breakfast table, and I stood right in front of her and said, 'Remember that this is my week to host poker.'" He turned back to Christy and said, "Remember?" Christy stared at him stone-faced, turned to me, and said very matter of factly, "He never told me."

Josh looked at me and asked, "Why? Why does this sort of thing keep happening?" In an effort to put forgetfulness in its proper context, I explained to Josh, as I often explain to non-ADHD partners, that it's not unusual for a partner with ADHD to forget—a lot—because ADHD is neurobiological in origin and affects the part of the brain that is responsible for staying focused, sustaining effort, managing emotions, and accessing working memory (that is, remembering). This explanation was little consolation to Josh, who had to cancel his poker night at the last minute, but it is exceptionally important for the non-ADHD partner to always remember that, due to the neurobiological nature of ADHD, there is a tendency for the ADHD partner to forget; in fact it seems to be the norm rather than the exception. The ADHD partner does not mean to forget and doesn't do it on purpose. Josh needed to stay mindful of this and also fine-tune his system for telling Christy about his plans. I suggested that he always use some method of follow-up if there is something that he wants Christy to remember:

- Brightly colored sticky notes placed in her calendar or on the steering wheel of her car will capture her attention so that she has a better chance of remembering the information.

- Sending an e-mail or text message is a fast and efficient way to remind your partner of something, but always include a request for acknowledgment of the message. Without acknowledgment a text message or e-mail can be quickly forgotten. It would be a good idea to always end the e-mail or text message with: "Can you let me know that you got this?" Without any acknowledgment, you cannot assume that your partner will remember.

As far as the poker party incident, I encouraged Josh to let it go, chalk it up to experience, and intend to do things differently in the future.

Being Lured from Conversations by a Wandering Mind

You may have seen the silly T-shirt that has this saying on the front: "Some say I have ADHD, but they don't under—hey, look! A squirrel!" This joke summarizes a common habit the person with ADHD exhibits, which is that his mind gets distracted by something and his attention leaves the conversation. Our world today is full of stimuli that create distraction—even to someone without ADHD, but pretty much everything has the ability to distract the ADHD brain away from a conversation: it might be something or someone passing by, it might be a noise, or it can even be a squirrel. The widespread use of electronic devices seems to provide the greatest opportunity for distraction for someone with ADHD. Computers, a thousand cable television channels, gaming mechanisms, handheld devices—all can offer hours and hours of colorful, interesting activity and provide plenty of opportunity to get distracted. But cell phone use seems to get the biggest moans and grumbles from my non-ADHD partners, especially smartphones, which not only offer texting but also allow the user to send and receive e-mails.

One of my non-ADHD clients was tired of losing his partner's attention, in general, and especially frustrated with her cell phone use, so they set up some rules to address her inattention. He explained their new arrangement this way: "I've promised not to get mad when I notice that her mind has wandered and she isn't paying attention to what I'm saying. I give her a chance to refocus and listen a second time. I used to get irritated and upset, and just drop whatever I was trying to say, but I don't do that anymore. I just go ahead and repeat the story or joke and don't get angry about it. Also, we have a hard-and-fast rule: she can't use her cell phone on date night—from the time we get in the car until we arrive home: no calls, texting, or checking e-mail. I know that this is exceptionally hard for her, but there are no exceptions." They are both fully aware of how her ADHD affects their relationship, especially her tendency to get distracted. Rather than allowing anger and defensiveness to take up their time together, they opted to look for a solution that would bring relief to the problem, and this agreement seems to work for them.

Getting distracted by outside stimuli is a common problem for someone with ADHD, but the ADHD brain can leave a conversation even if there isn't anything to distract it, due to *understimulation*. The problem with an understimulated brain is that despite efforts to concentrate on the conversation, the ability to stay focused fades away. Naturally the brain starts to seek something interesting, and if it can't find it in an outside source—something or someone—it might go to an internal source, such as daydreaming or becoming "lost in thought." During a therapy session I am very alert to the possibility of my ADHD client's mind going somewhere else in the middle of our conversation, and I've become skillful at noticing it as it happens. Even though my client may be nodding his head in agreement and saying, "Uh-huh," I observe his eyes slowly glazing over and then watch as his attention wanders away to a different part of the room. I realize that he isn't listening to anything I am saying, so I often stop at that point and comment on what I am experiencing by asking, "What were you just thinking about?" I'll hear something like "I was just thinking about going to the Dodger game on Friday" or "I was just thinking how your desk reminds me of a desk I had at my last job." I've learned to not take it personally, because I understand that it isn't unusual for the ADHD brain to feel understimulated and that, when the ADHD brain feels that way, the tendency will be for it to go somewhere else—anywhere else—to find something stimulating.

Consider this situation: you are having a conversation with your partner who has ADHD about, say, the electric bill, the kids needing new shoes, or news from your family back in Michigan. You observe the same thing that I see happen: the eyes glaze over and wander away to a different part of the room or out the window. As this situation is repeated over time, your assumption may be that, because your partner doesn't seem to be listening, she is rude and doesn't care for you. It's not necessarily true; it could be that her ADHD brain needs to be stimulated in order to pay attention, and unfortunately, conversations about bills, kids' shoes, or your family generally don't supply enough of it. Consequently you experience your partner leaving the conversation and you possibly feel offended. Perhaps you could offset any hurt feelings if you pointed out to your partner what you were noticing, shared with your partner how you felt disrespected and unimportant when it happened, and suggested that, together, you come up with a signal or a phrase that would alert her when you notice her leaving the conversation. My client would say to his partner, "Okay, honey, let's reset," and that was their arrangement to let her know that he noticed she had stopped paying attention to what he was saying. She agreed that she would not become defensive whenever he said, "Let's reset," and would make a renewed effort to stay in the conversation.

Speaking Out Impulsively

A person with ADHD is generally unaware of how he presents in public, that is, how others might perceive him when he does or says certain things. This is especially true with impulsively spoken words, which can catch others off guard and create uncomfortable situations. A person with ADHD can be pretty clueless as to what he has said. Joanne dreaded going to a social event, or any kind of event for that matter, with her husband, Victor, who had ADHD. He had a habit of blurting out inappropriate comments or questions to friends and even to strangers. Once, after their son's soccer game, a group of parents was standing around chatting. Victor asked one female parent why she had put on so much weight lately. After a moment of stunned silence, everyone quietly walked away. Victor turned to Joanne and innocently asked, "What did I do? All I did was ask a question."

Once again we can look to the brain for an explanation. The specific area of the brain that controls impulsivity is thought to be affected by the neurobiological impairment attributed to ADHD, and the result is that there is less ability to hold back impulsive speech. Here is a simple explanation that I often use for what's going on: Everyone has the potential to speak their thoughts out loud, but imagine that inside every brain, there is a little door that serves to guard against saying something too quickly. If the door is functioning well, it stays tightly shut and locked until the brain takes a moment to judge whether or not releasing the thought or question would be appropriate or wise, considering the circumstances. A person with ADHD has a door in the brain, too, but the door isn't functioning properly: the lock is broken because of ADHD, so there is less ability to keep the door tightly shut long enough to consider the thought or question before releasing it. As Joanne said to me, "Victor thinks it and says it; there seems to be nothing in between." Joanne has learned to handle embarrassing social situations with humor and may make a comment about how much Victor likes the taste of shoe leather, but she still experiences some level of anxiety when they go out because she is never sure what he might say. Fortunately, Joanne's awareness of her partner's ADHD has helped her to feel confident that she "can be okay without everything actually being okay," which is an important thing to remember.

Impulsive language due to ADHD might present social difficulties that create embarrassment for you, but it can be quite upsetting when it is aimed at you. Your partner may tend to interrupt you and not let you finish what you want to communicate. Warren would consistently interrupt and speak over his wife in our sessions. Her frustration was evident on her face each time he jumped in without allowing her to finish a sentence. When I pointed out to him that he continually interrupted his wife, he was surprised and got a little defensive with me. But Warren loved his wife and wanted their relationship to be better, so he was able to set aside his need to defend himself, and agreed that they needed to find a way to make this situation better. They came up with a hand signal: she would put her index finger to her nose, which would signal Warren that he had just interrupted her. Having a visual reminder can be helpful for an ADHD partner.

The greatest damage created by impulsive language is when your ADHD partner says hurtful things to you or hurls personal insults at you. While it usually occurs only during times of great stress or crisis, it doesn't erase the resulting injury. There is no excuse for this type of behavior, and it should not be tolerated. Verbally abusive relationships are extremely destructive. If verbal abuse from your ADHD partner is a chronic problem and there is no acknowledgment or effort to change, you may need to make some difficult decisions. It would be best to seek counseling with someone whom you can trust and who can help you sort out your situation.

Acting Impulsively

Just as ADHD can cause a person to say something before thinking, it can also cause someone to do first and think later. If your partner makes a quick decision at the end of the day to go out with buddies instead of coming home, it will probably bother you, and if it becomes a persistent pattern, there will be big problems in your relationship. If your partner has a habit of going on shopping sprees without consulting you, you might get very upset. The impulsive behavior doesn't have to be extreme or involve a lot of money to be problematic. Impulsive behavior comes across as selfishness and makes a person appear to be self-centered. If you feel that your partner is concerned about only her needs and wants, and acts on them impulsively, over time you may begin to feel that your needs and wants are less important in the relationship.

• Audrey

Audrey had a real problem with impulsive behavior, and her relationship with her partner, Joel, was suffering because of it. She was extremely creative, and one way she expressed her creativity was to do crafts—of any kind. But there were a couple of problems with Audrey's crafting. She would get a great idea from a magazine and then go out and buy everything she needed for the project, which meant outspending her budget. And then she would lay everything out on the dining room table while figuring out how to make the item look as it did in the magazine. When her attempts failed, which they often did, she got quickly bored with the project, and then another crafty thing would catch her eye. Impulsively, off she would go to buy all of the materials, and the whole thing would happen all over again. One week it would be a beading project, and the next it would be refurbishing furniture. Her husband, besides being bothered by the excess expenses, felt as if her impulsive need to do her craft projects took precedence over him. He felt tired of "competing with beads and fabrics," as he said. Audrey and Joel's relationship got worse: he would erupt in a rage, tell her that she could not spend one more penny on a craft idea, and threaten to throw everything out. Audrey would react strongly, and another fight would ensue. To expect Audrey to give up crafting and get rid of all of her supplies was unreasonable in light of her ADHD. But out of his frustration, Joel's tolerance level had fallen to zero, rendering him totally inflexible.

As the non-ADHD partner, you will find it important to factor impulsivity into your relationship. Once everything calmed down, Joel realized that part of his partner's ADHD manifestation was, and would always be, impulsive acts. With humor, he decided to be grateful that she liked crafts rather than five-hundred-dollar shoes! Although it took some effort, Audrey and Joel found a compromise: they created a small craft nook in their garage. Because she didn't have as much room, Audrey agreed to limit the amount of supplies she bought. And Joel agreed that if she kept all of her supplies there, instead of on the dining room table, he would not complain and might even learn to appreciate her creativity, which he had lost the ability to do along the way.

Poor Time Management: Always Late and Leaving Things until the Last Minute

This double-whammy complaint, which manifests as chronic tardiness, failure to factor in time properly, and leaving things until the last minute, could possibly be the biggest complaint I hear. Your ADHD partner doesn't think it's a big deal, right? He might say, "What's so awful about being a little late?" But chronic lateness in a relationship tends to take on a life of its own after a while. The non-ADHD partner gets weary of waiting around for the ADHD partner to get ready or show up. She may feel that her ADHD partner does not respect her time and preferences. Over time it is a struggle not to take it personally.

Because the ADHD partner treats time as fluid rather than finite, she tends to underestimate how much time it takes to do things or to get somewhere. I learned early on in my career about the fluid-versus-finite concept of time for the person with ADHD. A client with ADHD who had a standing appointment every Thursday at 10:00 a.m. was consistently ten to fifteen minutes late every week. We discussed it, and I decided to move the appointment to 10:30, thinking that she needed more time in the morning. But then she consistently showed up at 10:45! She truly wanted to be on time: she wasn't being resistant at all. But it seemed that even if she was ready to leave on time, she was still late because she tended to do "just one more thing" before leaving. Here is the irony of the "just one more thing" trap: it's never anything so important that it couldn't be done later. For this client, "just one more thing" was something like cleaning out her makeup drawer, printing an article she had found online, or moving around some of the plants on her patio. Before she knew it, she had used up any time that would have allowed her to arrive at our appointment on time.

Kenneth complained to me that his wife, Abby, was never on time. He felt that she was inconsiderate of his time and effort to be ready, and he often found himself angry and upset with her. When Abby was late, it wasn't because a crisis or catastrophe had occurred, but more often because she fell into the "just one more thing" trap. She felt that there was always time to do just one more thing before leaving. The problem was that she always misjudged how long it would take her to do that one last thing, which consequently caused them to be late.

Additionally, the "just one more thing" trap never leaves room for error, such as lost keys, bad traffic, or other things that always need to be factored in. Kenneth finally came to terms with Abby's time management issues, and rather than let himself consistently become impatient and upset, he decided that sometimes, if it was appropriate, he would leave on his own and meet her at their destination, or he would engage in a pleasurable activity, such as a crossword puzzle, while waiting.

When I work on time management issues with clients who have ADHD, I point out to them that time is finite, just like money, and illustrate it this way: I spread out some play money all over the table in my office and say, "If you go into the grocery store and have fifteen one-dollar bills to spend, you can't spend twenty-five or thirty. It just doesn't work that way. Please show me how I can get twenty-five dollars out of the fifteen I have here." Then I ask them to figure out how many "time dollars" are needed to complete their daily tasks: getting ready in the morning, driving to work or to the kids' school, preparing meals, and so on. This visual demonstration helps to conceptualize time as a concrete commodity, not something that has no end.

Procrastination

Some non-ADHD partners describe their ADHD partners' procrastination as "circling before landing." All of us put things off from time to time, but people with ADHD seem to have an exceptionally hard time getting started on something (unless they want to). It's important to understand that the ADHD brain needs to be stimulated in order to be motivated to get something done. None of us procrastinates when there is something we want to do. Does your partner with ADHD, if he is male and sports minded, procrastinate about getting involved in a sports event? Charlotte had tried everything, but could not get her partner to agree to complete the planting in their backyard, even though summer was approaching. But he was up at the crack of dawn and out the door to stand in line for playoff tickets. Procrastination is more likely to show up when there is something to do that is either unpleasant or unfulfilling. The ADHD brain tends to avoid chores, tasks, or activities that are unpleasant or unfulfilling, because they do not provide enough stimulation to properly activate the brain.

When an ADHD partner's procrastination affects a mutually shared plan or goal, it can create quite a bit of relational distress. Every year Rosa dreaded tax season because her partner, Daniel, who had ADHD, would always put his tax preparation off until the last minute. She began fretting in January, reminding Daniel about taxes right after the start of the new year, even though they had several months to go. She would gather up all of her information and have it ready for filing, but Daniel kept putting his part off. Even more frustrating for Rosa, she would see him make some effort along the way, but before too long, the boring and tedious task would be pushed aside and he would go off and do something less important but more stimulating to him. This dynamic caused quite a bit of misery for them in their relationship. Rosa would remind and remind, then complain and get angry. Daniel called her a nag and got angry too.

Arnold was frustrated every year with his ADHD partner's procrastination too. He and Marjorie took a vacation every summer to the family lake house. It was something that he looked forward to, and he thought Marjorie did too. But every year, Marjorie would procrastinate and wait to pack her suitcases until the night before they were to leave. Leaving packing to the last minute presented another set of problems, because Marjorie had difficulty deciding what to take and often discovered, when it was too late to go to a store, that she didn't have something she felt she needed. As the pressure built, Marjorie would get edgy and irritable, and a big blowout would occur. As a result they would depart for their trip barely speaking to each other. He was tired of this dynamic and felt that her procrastination meant she didn't care enough about him.

Both of these couples were very unhappy with how the ADHD symptom of procrastination concerning important tasks was creating such conflict in their relationships. They decided to work very hard to find other ways to address their situations. For Rosa and Daniel, it meant finding a reliable bookkeeper to come to their house once a month and keep Daniel's finances current. Marjorie decided to engage the services of a professional organizer to help her prepare for her trip.

Chronic Moodiness

While not an official part of an ADHD diagnosis, excessive mood reactivity is very common in ADHD (Feifel and MacDonald 2008). Moodiness is a hard dynamic to live with and can greatly affect the stability of a relationship.

• Charles

Charles was not diagnosed with ADHD until he was an adult. Throughout his childhood, he knew that something was not right and, consequently, grew up feeling that he couldn't perform as well as others. As a young adult, he continued to have these feelings and also felt that he would never be able to achieve success, that he was doomed to failure. As his feelings of failure grew, he also experienced a poor sense of self. All of these negative feelings that he had felt for so many years became a part of his identity, and consequently Charles carried a substantial amount of guilt and shame about himself all the time.

Interestingly, Charles had found a niche occupation and done well for himself. So from the outside, Charles looked very successful and appeared to "have it all." But if even one small thing went wrong during the course of a day, it affected how he thought about himself, bringing up the uncomfortable but all too familiar feelings of guilt and shame. Then his mood would change due to all of the internalized negative feelings that had become a part of what he believed about himself: *I'm a screwup. I'm stupid.* Once his partner became aware of how ADHD was negatively affecting his self-talk, she was able to feel more empathic and not be so affected by his moodiness.

Constant distractibility can create moodiness. Well-made plans are subverted by something less important, causing emotional stress and strain. Annette noticed that her partner would go out to the garage on Saturday mornings, all set to tackle a chore, and exhibit a noticeably different mood by the time afternoon came around. If he was cheerful and in good spirits at breakfast, he would become short tempered and prickly by four. It turned out that he would initially get distracted with his tools and projects in the garage, but in the afternoon it would dawn on him that he couldn't finish his intended task. At that point his ADHD-driven negative self-talk would take over and convince him that he couldn't accomplish anything at all. Unaware of what was underlying his changed mood, he directed his irritability at Annette, which caused considerable conflict in their relationship because Annette had done nothing to contribute to his bad mood. She couldn't imagine what had happened in such a short time. When they came to realize that he had ADHD, they understood that his moodiness was probably caused by his inability to stay on the task at hand and his resulting frustration was misdirected at Annette. As Annette realized the reason for his mood shift, she was able to understand how hard it must be for someone who has ADHD to deal with that kind of frustration.

All of these complaints—checking out of a conversation, putting important things off due to distractibility, poor time management, and moodiness—usually aren't deal breakers on their own. Very few people divorce their partners citing poor time management as the reason. Yet, over time, when these ADHD symptoms are actively played out in the relational dimension, they tend to erode relational harmony. Feelings change, resentment and negativity set in, and that's when couples find that the relationship is in trouble. It's important for the non-ADHD partner to always keep in mind that ADHD causes these unusual behaviors and that if the ADHD partner could make consistent changes, things would be different. A therapist or counselor who understands how ADHD can affect a relationship could help you and your partner with ADHD sort all of this out.

Sexual Difficulties

A satisfying sexual relationship comprises many components. Each partner must be mentally, emotionally, and physically engaged to achieve mutual satisfaction. All of the debilitating factors involved with ADHD—distractibility, impulsivity, and restlessness—come into play significantly where sex is concerned, and sexual frustration is very common in relationships involving a partner with ADHD.

DISTRACTIBILITY DURING SEX

To please a partner sexually, you must give great attention to the immediate situation, not to what's going on in the environment. Any type of disruption can cause a partner with ADHD to get distracted and lose focus. Many non-ADHD partners complain that in order for their partners to be able to fully engage in sex, there can be no distractions present: no candles causing flickering light on the wall, no music playing, and no sex talk during lovemaking. Although a quiet environment might help sex to happen without interruption, the sex might not be as mutually satisfying as it could be.

IMPULSIVITY CONCERNING SEX

Due to impulsivity, a partner with ADHD may want to have sex at what might seem to be inappropriate times. Keep in mind that when impulsive thoughts pop into the ADHD mind, very little filtering occurs. The non-ADHD partner, who is more aware of the surroundings and has a better sense of appropriateness, may become the gatekeeper for sex, the one who decides when it can happen. The partner with ADHD who impulsively approaches the non-ADHD partner for sex may be rejected often, which can create offense. The reality is that the non-ADHD partner may be very interested in sex, but because of the inappropriate timing, it may appear that the non-ADHD partner is not into it as much as the ADHD partner is.

Viewing pornography can also be an outgrowth of impulsive behavior. Pornography is easily accessed and readily available. While viewing pornography may not be a problem for some couples—some watch it together to enhance their lovemaking—for many it crosses personal boundaries and can interfere with the relationship. It's important to remember that an ADHD partner's viewing of pornography doesn't necessarily mean that he has a sexual problem or doesn't desire his partner; it may simply be that he has engaged in an impulsive act due to ADHD. But if pornography is used in place of true sexual intimacy, if it takes up the majority of your partner's free time or steps into inappropriate areas, there could be other issues that are separate from ADHD impulsivity and may require a more serious assessment.

RESTLESSNESS INITIATING SEX

Restlessness or boredom can be problematic for a couple's sexual relationship and can manifest in different ways for different people. Norma thought her husband was a sex addict. It didn't matter what tasks Norma had to do or what her responsibilities were; he always wanted and expected sex. But what really happened was that whenever he got bored or didn't have anything to do, his mind went to sex. Since he had ADHD, he felt bored a lot. Although she hated to do so, Norma had to say no often, which made her husband angry. He thought she didn't care for him, because if she did, she would want to have sex as often as he did. Norma began to dread the hour when he returned from work, because she knew the subject would come up during the course of an evening. Neither partner realized that his sexual appetite was due, in part, to boredom and restlessness caused by ADHD.

Lisa and Patrick's sexual relationship was in trouble due to Patrick's restlessness from ADHD. Lisa was reluctant to have sex at all with Patrick anymore. She said that in the beginning of their relationship, they had experienced a very healthy and mutually satisfying sex life. But little by little, Patrick had begun to express a desire for more varied sexual experiences. That was fine with Lisa; she was not opposed to sexual experimentation. But nothing ever seemed to be enough for Patrick. Patrick wanted not only frequent sex, but also longer, more intense, or more explosive experiences than the time before, or else he expressed disappointment. He accused Lisa of not being interested in him anymore. Lisa felt that his expectations were far too unreasonable for the reality of their lives. They both worked demanding jobs, and they had small children. She said she wasn't always physically and emotionally available for Patrick's "sexual Olympics," as she called it. As they both came to understand how ADHD can affect a couple's sexual relationship, they realized that Patrick desired lots of sexual fireworks for stimulation to offset his feelings of boredom or restlessness.

As we have seen in this chapter, the challenges of being in and staying in a relationship show up in spades when ADHD is involved. There may be problems with communication and social skills due to impulsivity and distractibility. Your partner with ADHD might get bored with a conversation and change the subject or walk away, possibly leading you to think that she is "not into you" or, worse, that she is totally rude and uncaring. And partners with ADHD tend to forget things a lot. Forgetting to stop by the grocery to pick up a carton of milk, while annoying, isn't a big deal, but when birthdays and anniversaries are forgotten, the stakes get higher. And, as we have found, restlessness can create sexual boredom, leading a partner to demand more and more or perhaps to look outside the relationship for satisfaction.

I often advise my non-ADHD clients to imagine what it would be like to have ADHD, to "walk a mile" in their partners' shoes. By staying aware and consistently mindful of ADHD, you can avoid a lot of relational pain and suffering. Here is some shared wisdom from some non-ADHD partners about how they handle their feelings and emotions as they try to understand ADHD and how it affects their partners:

- "I try to remind myself that he really does have trouble focusing. Usually, when he gets home at the end of his workday, it's important for me to remember that because he has focused all day on work tasks, his 'focus meter' needs a rest. I wait for a better time to try to engage with him when I need him to focus on something."

- "Although it's very hard for me, I need to adjust my expectations. That allows me to be better at caring for my wife, who has ADHD."

- "I've learned that he has struggled with 'messing up' his whole life, and that helps me to be more understanding about what he goes through on a day-to-day basis."

- "Continuing to research and understand ADHD has helped me to be more empathic and to avoid interpreting all of his actions in a negative manner. I now understand that so much of his behavior is not aimed at hurting me; rather he is just very self-focused due to ADHD."

CHAPTER 5

The Emotional Dimension

The day-to-day disturbances of ADHD—distractibility, restlessness, procrastination, forgetfulness—can cause your partner with ADHD to develop emotional difficulties. Although you may not be aware of it, your partner constantly struggles to stay focused by trying to remember what others have said, remain on task, stay attentive to details, and be mindful of her own words and actions. The constant frustration that your partner may experience from such difficulties can be emotionally debilitating and can reveal itself in several different ways.

Inaccurate Self-Assessment

For someone with ADHD, at the core of the emotional dimension is a tendency to hold an inaccurate self-image that can lead to a negative sense of worth because of consistently problematic ADHD behaviors: forgetfulness, poor time management, distractibility, procrastination, and lack of follow-through. More often than not, parents, teachers, coaches, employers, and so on reinforced this negative sense of self through the years. Unfortunately, making someone with ADHD feel bad for shortcomings that he has little control over only serves to further reinforce his negative beliefs about himself.

• Natalie

A lovely woman who was very talented and creative, Natalie, a client with ADHD, had a very poor sense of self-worth. As a child, she regularly had been lectured for hours (literally) about how bad she was because she had forgotten to do some chore. Every week her parents would verbally rattle off a list of tasks to be performed. Her undiagnosed and untreated ADHD interfered with her ability to remember their chore list, so she almost always forgot at least one thing and, more often, forgot everything past the first item on the list. Every Saturday afternoon she dreaded the shaming lecture that would come the moment her parents would discover what she had forgotten. Natalie's poor self-image followed her into her adult life. Her automatic response to every mistake she made as an adult was *I'm such a loser*, which is how she had been made to feel about herself as a child. It took a long time for her to work through her negative view of herself, but understanding that it was ADHD that caused her inability to remember was immensely helpful.

However, it's not uncommon to get another, very different reaction. Your partner may have trouble accepting responsibility for the times when his ADHD behavior causes problems. Rather than an automatic *I'm such a loser* response, like Natalie had, your partner may resist accepting accountability for shortcomings and may respond with something more like: "I didn't do anything wrong," blaming someone or something else for his mistakes. Angela's husband, Christopher, who refused to accept his ADHD diagnosis, illustrates this predicament well.

• Angela and Christopher

Christopher planned a wonderful birthday for their young teenage daughter, telling her he would hire a limousine and arrange for it to pick her and her friends up at school for a "night on the town" that included dinner and a movie. Christopher was to meet the limo at school and accompany the girls for the evening, and then bring them home for a sleepover that Angela, his wife, would oversee. Their daughter was over the moon with excitement, and there was much discussion at home as the day grew closer. The big day arrived, and at about four in the afternoon, Angela got a call from their daughter, asking if she had heard from Christopher, because the limo was there but her dad wasn't. Christopher never showed up. By six Angela had frantically called the local hospitals and law enforcement to see if Christopher had been in an auto accident. At six thirty Angela got a call from Christopher, and before she could say anything, he said, "Hey honey, I'm heading home and just wondered if you needed me to pick up anything."

Due to his ADHD, Christopher had forgotten this terrific special event that *he* had created and planned. At our next session, when I asked him about the forgotten birthday, he showed little remorse and, instead, gave an immediate and heated response. Leaning forward in a rather aggressive manner, he informed me that he was a very important businessman and was flooded every day with hundreds of decisions to make and things to do—and anyway, it wasn't his fault, because his assistant should have reminded him.

Both Natalie's and Christopher's responses represent the shame that arises when ADHD symptoms cause mistakes. Natalie would feel like and refer to herself as a "loser" because she had been programmed to regard herself as a bad person whenever she forgot things or messed up somehow. Christopher felt the same way, but would go on the defensive to protect himself from feeling bad about a mistake.

Rather than try to cheerlead your partner with ADHD through her negative self-statements or react negatively to defensive responses, which can be tiring and frustrating, keep in mind that your partner's negative sense of worth and significance was created way before you came along. Offer empathy, understanding, and kindness, and try to love your partner through difficult times.

Irritability

Along with a negative self-image, your ADHD partner's emotional responses can also result in an irritable mood. The emotional energy that is necessary to handle ADHD symptoms can result in a lowered tolerance for anything that is frustrating. As a result, you may notice that your partner is more irritable than usual and gets upset over little things that shouldn't ordinarily be problems. Or he may display a short fuse by verbally lashing out. His irritability can come about for no apparent reason; he may seem to be in a great frame of mind in the morning, but a downward swing soon occurs. And unfortunately, all of his emotional states can spill over into your relationship and affect you.

You are an eyewitness to your partner's struggles. You have a front-row seat to the consequences of her ADHD behavior and of her difficulty with staying on target. If you offer a helpful reminder or ask a question, you may get a hostile or resentful reaction because your partner may feel that her ADHD has been "exposed."

• Frank and Gina

I once counseled a couple named Frank and Gina. Gina had ADHD, inattentive type. Sometimes, when Frank would ask a question, such as "What time is dinner?" Gina would blow up at him. Because of her ADHD, she had trouble organizing her time and efforts, and was often very late in getting dinner to the table for the family. In this instance, when Frank asked her what time dinner would be, he really just wanted to know how much time he had to finish what he was doing. But Gina heard the question as a sharp reminder that she had, once again, failed to take care of her responsibilities, which in this case meant having dinner ready on time. The anger she expressed in response to Frank represented her negative feelings about her perceived failures. Whenever Gina lashed out at Frank, he felt ambushed and would then respond in anger himself, thus beginning a very unhealthy cycle of quarreling. Frank felt that there was never a good time to ask Gina about anything, and their communication had almost stopped completely.

I explained to both of them that Gina's irritability could be due to ADHD, specifically prompted by Frank's questions or comments, which reminded her that, once again, she had failed to stay on target. This explanation helped them to gain insight into why they consistently fought, and as a result, they were able to begin to work out a more effective way to avoid this toxic pattern in the future.

The irritability that seems to come out of nowhere is always surprising, and attempting to maintain a relationship with someone who is irritable is not pleasurable or satisfying. If you find yourself walking on eggshells when you are around your partner who has ADHD, just be aware that, regardless of how loving or caring you might behave, you may still serve as a reminder to your partner of his self-perceived shortcomings, and the possibility that you will be the recipient of your partner's emotional unrest is always present. Try not to take it personally. Dig deep within yourself and continue to find empathy for your partner by trying to understand how hard it can be for him to handle his struggles with ADHD.

Depression

One of the biggest complaints that people with ADHD have is difficulty in keeping up with life's challenges. Recently, a client with ADHD recalled a variety television show he had seen as a child, in which one of the acts involved a man who spun large plates on long sticks. The goal was to get about eight to ten plates spinning at the same time. Just as it seemed that all of the plates were spinning well, one plate would start to wobble and appear to be in danger of crashing to the ground. The entertainer would quickly run over and get the plate spinning again, but just as he resolved that situation—you guessed it—another plate at the other end of the line would begin to wobble, and so on and so on. My client said, "That has been my whole life! Just when everything seems to be under control, the potential for disaster occurs."

When a person with ADHD spends all of her time frantically trying to keep all of the plates spinning (fighting off distractibility, and staying focused and alert), she can become very frustrated. If your partner feels that, no matter what she does, she is unsuccessful at bringing about desired changes in her life, she may begin to feel worn out and eventually lose hope that life will ever be any different. Over time and with consistency, these general feelings of disappointment and discontent can develop into a deeper emotional issue, such as depression. It's not unusual for depression to exist along with ADHD; one disorder does not cancel out the other. In fact, in adult ADHD *comorbidity*—two or more disorders existing simultaneously—is common (Newcorn 2008).

When I treat someone who has depression, I tend to notice darker and more intense behaviors; for example, a person who might be content and positive under normal circumstances finds very little in life to be content and positive about when experiencing depression. If he is generally quiet and subdued, he will be even more so as he gets caught up in a downward spiral of negative thoughts. It's as though a small but very dark cloud has moved in and taken up residence above his head. Despite his best efforts to get it to leave, he can't make the cloud go away.

The negative beliefs that are never far away in ADHD—*I'm dumb, I'm lazy, I'm stupid, I'm bad*—are aggravated by a depressed state. These negative beliefs that are fueled by depression feed into your partner's personality and behaviors. If your partner with ADHD is depressed, you will notice a sadder demeanor and less inclination to do the things she used to enjoy: no joke will make her laugh, and she will ignore a favorite hobby that she previously enjoyed. Trying to cheer her up falls flat. She may lack an appetite regardless of how many enticing delicacies you offer. Or you may notice that she has developed an insatiable appetite, consuming voluminous amounts of junk food. She may drink more alcohol than usual, such as a whole bottle of wine in an evening, or she might disappear into a cloud of marijuana, which she previously used only recreationally. There may be a tendency for her to want to stay in bed all day, to pull the covers up and block out life regardless of planned activities or previous commitments. Or she may have more difficulty than usual going to sleep; perhaps you find her sitting in front of the television at 4:00 a.m. because she can't sleep.

Out of deep concern, you may point these things out to your partner and ask, "What's wrong? What's going on?" Chances are you won't get a definitive answer because, more often than not, your partner has little awareness of the depth of the depressed state that is fueling the behavior you are observing. What he does know is that something is different and not right; he just can't put his finger on it. He longs for a return to the way he "used to feel," but nothing seems to help. He is frustrated and unable to effect change. The very real danger with depression is that it has a tendency to continue spiraling downward and to become more severe and dangerous if left ignored and unattended.

The following symptoms of depression are based on the *DSM-IV-TR* (APA 2000):

- Decreased ability to concentrate or make decisions

- Diminished energy, tendency to be fatigued

- Feelings of inappropriate guilt or worthlessness

- Significantly reduced level of interest in or enjoyment from most or all activities

- Prolonged depressed mood

- Trouble falling asleep or staying asleep, or sleeping too much

- Observably agitated or slowed-down behavior

- Frequent thoughts of death or suicide, with or without a plan for carrying it out

- Considerable weight loss (5 percent or more in a month without dieting) or decrease in appetite, or considerable weight gain or increase in appetite

If you suspect that your partner is experiencing symptoms of depression, don't ignore the problem and hope it will just go away. Talk to her about what you have noticed. Express your concerns, tell her you love her, and offer to call her health care provider for an appointment.

Anxiety

People who have ADHD also commonly experience anxiety (Feifel and MacDonald 2008). Creating order and stability is challenging for someone with ADHD, so a considerable amount of anxious energy has to be created to stay on task and focused. A client with ADHD described her anxiety as feeling as if she were unexpectedly hit by handfuls of gravel all day long, with each little piece of gravel representing a new task or undertaking that required her attention and effort. Consequently, she spends a lot of time and emotional energy trying to figure out, or worrying about, how to handle all of the tasks that are thrown at her, and she feels constantly overwhelmed.

Mental energy spent worrying about everything, big or small, is another outcome of anxiety brought on by ADHD. Worry may feel as if it helps to keep the brain focused. For instance, your partner may feel that as long as he worries about something, he won't forget it. But worry has a negative effect, because it usually focuses on what could go wrong. Being consumed with anxious thoughts centering on what bad thing could happen in the future robs your partner of the ability to be fully present. The excessive worry and anxiety can create more mental distraction for your ADHD partner, resulting in his being even less emotionally available for you.

Anxious energy can drive not only thought processes but also behavior. The following common symptoms of anxiety, based on the *DSM-IV-TR* (APA 2000), illustrate how anxiety can affect both the mind and the body.

- Trouble sleeping

- Trouble concentrating

- Tense muscles

- Feeling wound up, tense, or restless

- Tendency to feel fatigued or worn out

One highly anxious client with ADHD usually arrives for her appointments breathless and scattered, with notes and papers falling out of her daily planner. She has trouble collecting her thoughts well enough for us to cover her concerns during the session and usually remembers something important as she walks out the door at the end. What I observe during the hour we meet once a week indicates how she lives her life, which she describes as always "playing catch-up." She says she always feels uneasy in her own skin, has trouble relaxing, can't organize a thought to save her life, and always feels physically exhausted from difficulty sleeping through the night.

Anxiety, like depression, tends to take on a life of its own, spilling over to affect others and making ADHD behaviors seem even more amplified. If your partner is anxious, he may have more difficulty than usual sitting still; he may appear even more jittery and nervous, and may have excessive trouble staying focused and alert. I have noticed that when I'm in a counseling session with an anxious person who has ADHD, I have to do a lot of inner self-talk to calm myself, because I can easily begin to feel anxious and jittery too. Many non-ADHD partners complain that they feel physically worn out by their partner's high level of anxiety. By managing to breathe deeply and evenly, and consciously relaxing the tension in my muscles, I am able to calm myself and become more centered during my sessions with an anxious client. If you find that you are absorbing your ADHD partner's anxiety in the same way, you might find it helpful to practice breathing and relaxation methods, such as the ones offered in chapter 6.

Besides affecting your relationship, anxiety can, over time, adversely affect your partner's health. There are indications that people with anxiety disorders are at greater risk of having heart attacks and other cardiovascular problems (Harvard Health Publications 2011). Panic attacks, a common manifestation of anxiety that mimics heart attack symptoms, can develop. The symptoms—sweating, racing heart, trouble breathing—create significant physical and emotional distress. The thoughts of an anxious person can become irrational and illogical; your partner may become immobilized from the effects of her anxiety and begin to withdraw from pleasurable activities or family obligations. At the very worst, agoraphobia can develop, which would cause your partner to leave home only with marked distress, or maybe not at all. Anxiety is a twenty-four-hour disorder, and it can affect every minute of your partner's life.

A person who has ADHD is particularly vulnerable to emotional disturbances for several reasons: he can feel that despite his determination and best efforts, things just don't turn out the way they should. He may have a habit of forgetting to do or say something, or may do or say something he shouldn't, so the specter of screwing up can be relentless and ongoing. In his mind the potential for another screwup is always a very real possibility. As a result, he may have established a negative opinion of himself and may express his emotions with too much anger or irritation. A relentless drive to be on constant alert to handle whatever comes along can create anxiety. Or he may get mentally and physically weary of the effort it takes for him to keep up, and therefore lose hope and fall into a depressed state.

All of the factors that show up in the emotional dimension of life can affect your relationship. Your partner's irritability can create conflict-ridden situations. Her anxiety can create serious health issues and add to an already distracted state of mind. And depression isolates your partner, creating an invisible and impenetrable barrier to intimacy. You may find yourself experiencing your own emotional distress as you try to manage the ups and downs of your partner's emotional states, which can cause you to feel exhausted and burned out.

Don't give up. There is help for all of the emotional problems your partner with ADHD experiences: medical management is very helpful for a depressed state or anxiety, and cognitive behavioral therapy has been shown to help smooth out moods and also assist in restructuring firmly entrenched negative self-opinions (Ramsay 2002).

PART 3

Strengthening Your Relationship

CHAPTER 6

Defusing Your Anger

The tears started pouring out as Melinda sat down on the couch in my office. When she was able to speak, her words rushed out in a cascade: "I'm so angry all of the time. I wake up angry, I stay angry all day, and I go to sleep angry." She continued with clenched fists, "I am not an angry person. I hate that I feel like this; it is so 'not me'!" When the tears subsided, I was able to get a clearer picture of why she was so emotional. Melinda was in a committed, long-term relationship with Joseph, with whom she had been for many years and had three children. After a recent cluster of job losses, Joseph had sought help to discover why he kept getting fired and, during the process, had been diagnosed with ADHD. Melinda had felt relieved initially. The diagnosis had helped her to understand so many things: why he had been let go from jobs for which he was highly qualified; why projects at home never got finished; why he was consistently late, even to important events; and why he had grown so distant and moody as life had become more complicated. Now she had a name for all of the things that caused her frustration.

As Melinda had learned about the symptoms of ADHD and discovered that effective treatment was available for it, she had felt hopeful for the first time in years and believed that things would get better. Her anger toward Joseph had subsided significantly. But Joseph's reaction was different. He was not thrilled with the diagnosis and was very reluctant to admit that he had "something wrong" with him, as he had put it. Consequently, he was resistant to treatment, and the problems surrounding his ADHD symptoms continued. Melinda's initial enthusiasm and optimism faded away, and her anger returned stronger than ever.

Melinda's statement, "I am not an angry person," was true. She admitted that she hardly ever felt angry, except when it came to Joseph, and added that no one else whom she knew would characterize her as an angry person. Melinda's situation is not unusual at all. Many non-ADHD partners who are calm and even-tempered find themselves engulfed in strong feelings of anger that have evolved from the frustration of dealing with a partner's ADHD.

The Effects of Anger

Anger that is born of frustration undermines the ability to process thoughts and emotions in a rational manner. It distorts perceptions and limits your ability to focus on reality. It curtails hope, potentially brings despair, and consumes both mind and spirit, often defining a person's identity. Anger creates barriers to new solutions, to better outcomes, and to the future.

Anger also has a powerful physical effect. It signals to the body that something is wrong, and the body snaps to attention and responds as though it needs to guard against a potential threat. So while you may be feeling anger toward your partner with ADHD because she has forgotten to pick up the kids from school again, your body doesn't know the difference between anger at her forgetfulness and anger that could be signaling a dangerous situation. Because of this warning system, the body springs into action, thinking it needs to protect and defend. The physical reaction to anger is quite amazing. Your body thinks it might need to make a quick getaway, so the following reactions occur:

- Brain chemicals are released that cause a quick burst of energy.

- The pancreas begins to control sugar balance to have energy for action.

- Your muscles become very tight and tense.

- Your heart rate goes up: 180 beats per minute versus a regular rate of 80 beats per minute.

- Your blood pressure rises: 220 over 130 or higher versus 120 over 80.

- Your external arteries constrict.

- Your pupils dilate.

- Your breathing pattern quickens to get more oxygen into your body.

- Blood flow increases to your extremities.

- Chemicals are released to clot the blood in case there is an injury.

Even more amazing, all of this happens instinctively, without any conscious thought given to the situation at hand. Because this happens involuntarily, it is extremely important to get a handle on your anger, because the repetitive wear and tear on your body and its metabolism can be disastrous. Long-term effects of anger can take a huge toll on the body. Some of the consequences associated with anger are:

- High blood pressure

- Tension headaches and migraines due to muscle spasms in the neck and head

- Insomnia

- Risk of heart attack or stroke owing to chemicals that are released to clot the blood (a clot can pass through the blood vessels to the brain or heart)

- Ulcers resulting from excess stomach acidity induced by stress

- Flare-ups of irritable bowel syndrome (IBS)

- Heightened sensitivity to noise, light, smell, and even touch

- Frequent colds and influenza, infections, asthma attacks, and flare-ups of skin diseases

- Diseases like arthritis caused by long-term hormonal imbalances that can affect the immune system

- Overeating, smoking, excessive drinking

- Higher risk of depression (which can trigger even more anger)

Furthermore, the body doesn't automatically relax once anger has subsided. Once aroused, your nervous system has difficulty calming down and can stay on alert for many hours. During the cool-down period, you can get angered again very easily and even continue to have harsh responses to minor issues. Melinda noticed that her kids would suddenly and mysteriously disappear after one of her arguments with her husband over ADHD issues. On reflection, she realized that during her cool-down period, she had been blowing up at the kids over small things that ordinarily did not bother her.

The Function of Anger

One way to defuse anger is to understand where it comes from and how it develops. It has been said that anger is a secondary emotion, that it masks other emotions, such as feelings of helplessness or vulnerability. If so, then anger has what is called *secondary gain*, which means that there is some benefit to the anger. Although it's hard to believe that anger could provide any benefit, viewing it as a secondary emotion can provide some sense of power as you realize that anger can serve as protection from frightening and upsetting core feelings. Melinda began to understand that her anger at Joseph was really covering her own feelings of fear about the future (vulnerability) and about her inability to control the consequences of her husband's behavior (helplessness). She was scared that if Joseph didn't take care of things, it would negatively affect the welfare of the family. Despite the fact that she worked part-time, Melinda didn't have the income-earning potential that Joseph had, so she was very frightened of what could happen. Although she wasn't aware of it, at least in the moment when Joseph's ADHD behavior triggered her fears of the future, her angry feelings did help to protect her from feeling helpless and completely vulnerable.

EXERCISE 6.1 ANGER JOURNAL

Is it possible that your anger is masking feelings of helplessness and vulnerability? By creating an anger journal, you will be able to track your anger and understand its function. Take a piece of paper or a notebook, or a laptop computer and do the following:

1. Make an entry date: the date and time you felt angry toward your partner who has ADHD.

2. List the event: describe what happened to make you feel angry.

3. Rate your anger on a scale of 1 to 5, in which 1 means not very angry at all and 5 means out-of-control anger.

4. Recall how your body felt. Describe your breathing pattern, your muscle tension, your heart rate, and so on.

5. Try to remember what you were thinking as you got angry, and write that down.

6. Record what action you took. What exactly did you do or say when you were angry?

7. Meditate on your anger for the purpose of discovering what the core feeling might have been.

Melinda's anger journal noted her feelings of anger at Joseph for being chronically late for work from failing to wake up on time. Melinda's first response to the last question was that she was angry because she was frustrated. While her frustration was understandable, I asked her to go further in investigating her feelings. She collapsed in another heap of tears when she realized how scared she was about the future: if Joseph was late to work too many times, his boss might fire him and then he might not be able to find another job quickly. These thoughts led her to worry about where and how they would live: how would they be able to afford their car, pay rent, and buy food and clothing for the kids? At her core, she felt very frightened. Melinda's anger was real, understandable, and justified, but it had gotten the best of her. When she realized that fear, along with feelings of hopelessness and vulnerability, were really fueling her anger, she was able to start to control it better.

Anger as a Grief Response

Anger can also be understood in another context: as a reaction to loss. During the course of our lives, we experience many types of losses, both concrete and abstract. *Concrete losses*, for instance, take the form of something real and tangible: the death of a loved one, a divorce, or losing a job or career. Less obvious, yet equally significant, are *abstract losses*. An abstract loss is usually centered on the loss of an expectation or an ideal that we have carried in our minds and hearts for a long time. Abstract losses aren't usually recognized as a loss or given much significance, because these types of losses aren't as easy to identify. Someone who experiences an abstract loss is often left to try to figure it out all alone, with very little understanding or support from family or friends.

A natural reaction to any loss, whether it is concrete or abstract, is grieving. Grieving begins when someone or something we care about is lost to us. It is widely acknowledged that there are several stages of grief that we experience in reaction to a loss. The most widely understood and accepted stage of grief is sadness. It's common to feel sad and down when a loss occurs. Another significant stage of grief is anger. But because people don't understand that anger is a strong component of grief, most people feel quite uncomfortable and perplexed when anger flares up in reaction to a loss. Healthy grieving runs its course when each stage of grief, including anger, is properly acknowledged and allowed to be experienced. But because an angry response to grief can be so uncomfortable and misunderstood, you may not recognize it as an appropriate response and consequently may not process it appropriately. When this grieving process is inhibited, a person can get stuck in the anger stage of grief, feeling angry most of the time.

Whenever I counsel non-ADHD partners who complain about feeling angry all the time, I help them to explore any unresolved grief due to lost expectations about the relationship. I explain that at the beginning of a relationship, there is hope and a vision for a partnership that will be enjoyable, mutually satisfying, and fulfilling. Even with an awareness of personal differences, the expectation is that both partners will use individual strengths and abilities to contribute to the relationship in a positive way, thus creating respect. But over time, ADHD behaviors can create problems that can influence the relationship in a negative way: procrastination, poor time management, distractibility, and moodiness, to mention a few. The dream of a relationship characterized by enjoyment, satisfaction, and fulfillment begins to erode.

At some point, the full awareness of the impact of your partner's ADHD hits: *This thing called ADHD is here to stay and will never go away; it will always have to be managed and treated, and will always affect our relationship in some way.* This awareness can be difficult enough to accept with mild to moderate ADHD symptoms and a compliant partner (one who agrees with the diagnosis and with treatment), but is made even harder if the ADHD symptoms are severe and there is no compliance. Along with the sobering awareness of having to deal with ADHD forever, you may be upset by the following realizations: *This isn't what I expected. This is not what I thought it would be. I didn't sign up for this!* As you come to terms with the full reality of what life is like and will continue to be like with your ADHD partner, you experience a loss, and a grief reaction is set in motion. You feel the anger associated with the grief response but don't understand it in the proper context. And without that understanding, the anger keeps playing out over and over again.

In our sessions, Melinda continued to process her anger to see if it could be further explained as unresolved grief. Her relationship with Joseph had begun with high hopes and expectations. She felt that she had chosen well: Joseph was a kind and gentle man with high values. She knew he was a little "quirky," as she called it, but overlooked this because she regarded him as so smart and talented. In the beginning they lived more or less autonomously: he did his thing, and she did hers; she worked, and so did he. She did notice that he was forgetful, but brushed it off as part of his quirkiness. There was also the matter of his job dissatisfaction; he had trouble keeping a job. He got bored, had trouble with a boss, or had difficulty with all of the rules and regulations. Melinda figured that Joseph just hadn't found his niche yet.

The real trouble began, as she recalled, when their first child was born. Joseph was thrilled with their son, but Melinda soon found that she couldn't depend on Joseph to help out very much. He never came home when he promised, because he waited until the end of the day to start the paperwork for his job. He would stay up too late to be of any help with nighttime feedings, because his computer games would mesmerize him. He lost his job when the baby was six months old because he was late too many times. Melinda was disappointed but figured that maybe this was just a hard transition for him. To take up the slack, Melinda took on part-time work, just to tide them over until Joseph found another job. At this point a new pattern began to develop in their relationship: little by little Joseph dropped responsibilities, and Melinda picked them up. It got worse with the birth of each child, because Melinda had to depend on Joseph even more than before. She was frustrated with the relationship and, from time to time, would "lose it" with him, erupting in angry outbursts. Joseph would promise to try harder and to pay more attention to Melinda's needs, but over time his effort would fade due to his undiagnosed and untreated ADHD, and the relationship fell back into the same dissatisfying pattern.

Then Joseph lost three jobs in a row, being fired at the end of each probationary period due to tardiness, inattention to details, and, in one instance, speaking rudely to a customer. Both he and Melinda thought it might be a good idea for him to see their doctor for a checkup, just in case there was something going on physically. During the course of Joseph's examination, after asking some questions, his doctor told Joseph that he suspected ADHD, and recommended a specialist. After an evaluation by the specialist, Joseph was diagnosed with ADHD, combined type, and medication and personal therapy were recommended. Joseph was doubtful about the diagnosis, since he had known some kids in school who had ADHD and "was nothing like them." He said, "How could he give me that diagnosis after spending only thirty minutes with me?" Joseph felt that all he needed was a less stressful job.

Melinda, in the meantime, had gone on a crash course to learn as much as she could about ADHD. She spent time online and read several books that explained ADHD in adults. As she learned, she shared the information with Joseph, hoping that it would help motivate him to get the appropriate treatment for his ADHD symptoms. The more he resisted, the angrier she became, until one day she thought to herself, *This just isn't working. I don't have to put up with this! I've sacrificed the best years of my life for him, and I'm done!* and began to make plans to leave Joseph. She was tired of being angry because things had not turned out as she had thought they would.

Prior to consulting with a divorce attorney, she decided it would be a good idea to get help for herself, and that's when she found herself in my office. I was able to help Melinda understand that, in essence, her anger was unresolved grief due to the loss of an ideal about her relationship with Joseph. Her initial hope and vision at the beginning of their relationship for an enjoyable, satisfying, and fulfilling partnership had faded away over time. She had given up on her expectations of her relationship with Joseph and was unknowingly grieving this loss. During the course of our therapy, she gave herself permission to actively grieve, and was able to finally accept the loss of her ideal and to accept her relationship with Joseph as it was. She reported that her seething anger had subsided and that she was no longer the angry person she used to be. Previously, any attempt to discuss ADHD with Joseph had resulted in angry exchanges and remarks. When Melinda's anger wasn't the central issue anymore, they were able to have some productive conversations about ADHD, and at last report, Joseph had begun to come around by stating that he would consider treatment.

If you think your anger could be the result of an unresolved loss in your life, then it is worth the time and effort to examine the history of your relationship with your partner who has ADHD. As difficult as it might be, try to remember what your hopes and aspirations were at the beginning of your relationship. Reflect on how the relationship may have changed due to your partner's ADHD. Consider what has been lost to you and to your relationship. Determine whether or not you are stuck in an anger cycle. If you find that this concept could be contributing to your anger, then give yourself permission to feel the feelings that are attached to grief, including disbelief, sadness, and anger. If you find that you stay angry, you may need help in this process. Enlist the aid of a wise counselor or therapist who can help you sort out your feelings and bring finality to your grieving process.

Recovering from Anger

Your anger may serve the purpose of protecting you from feeling helpless or vulnerable. Perhaps it is the result of unrecognized grief. Or it could be both, as it was with Melinda. As you endeavor to gain insight and awareness, here are some guidelines for better equipping yourself to handle your anger.

Externalize the ADHD

When you feel angry at your partner because of something she has or hasn't done, try to remember to tell yourself that ADHD is causing the behavior. Over time we tend to think of ADHD behavior as a character issue: *What kind of a person would treat another with so much disrespect!* Regardless of how it may appear, your partner who has ADHD is aware at some level of how the behaviors may be affecting your life, and she would like nothing better than to be rid of the problematic behaviors forever. So the next time you find yourself gritting your teeth because of something your partner with ADHD has done or said (or not done or said), rather than get angry at her, try to tell yourself, *There it goes again; that's the ADHD acting up.* Reminding yourself to externalize the ADHD behavior will transform it from a character issue into an impairment. Get mad at ADHD, not your partner.

The Importance of Daily Renewal

You need to take time to care for yourself and your emotional health. I recommend the following two exercises for this purpose.

EXERCISE 6.2 MINDFULNESS

Try doing a mindfulness exercise once a day. When you are angry, you are less likely to be mindful of the world around you. The result is that you spend a lot of mental energy thinking about the past and ruminating about what your partner with ADHD has done to make you angry. Mindfulness is designed to bring you into the present, to help you to be more aware and appreciative of what is going on around you. By spending only a few minutes each day meditating on your five senses, you can be more grounded in the present and better able to leave the past behind. It's a simple but effective exercise:

1. Find a comfortable, quiet place to lie down or sit.

2. Close your eyes and begin to concentrate on what you *hear*. For thirty to sixty seconds, shut out all the other senses and concentrate *only* on what you hear. Can you hear birds chirping that you were previously unaware of? If there is traffic outside, concentrate on the sounds of the traffic—not just as noise but also as individual sounds.

3. Continue to keep your eyes closed, but switch your concentration from what you hear to what you smell. Can you smell the soap you used when you bathed this morning? Are there any smells in the room that you didn't notice before? Remember to shut down all of the other senses as you concentrate on smell.

4. With your eyes still closed, leave the sense of smell and concentrate for thirty to sixty seconds on what you taste in your mouth. Can you still taste your morning coffee or the garlic from your pasta dinner the night before?

5. Next, shift to touch. With your eyes still shut, focus on what your body feels. How do your clothes feel as the fabric touches your body? Are your clothes loose or tight? How does the chair you are sitting on feel to your touch? Are you comfortable? Concentrate on the details of these sensations. Be totally aware of everything that touches your skin.

6. And last, open your eyes to concentrate on sight. Shut down all other senses and look around you; really look. Notice the colors and variations of colors that you see: the shadows, the shapes, and the lines. Concentrate only on sight for thirty to sixty seconds.

This simple mindfulness exercise is designed to raise your awareness of your surroundings in a new and different way. Taking a few minutes out of your day to practice this new discipline will help you to live more in the moment and, at least for a few minutes, to be able to step away from anger that is rooted in the past.

EXERCISE 6.3 EXAMEN OF CONSCIOUSNESS

This exercise—its origin dating back to the 1500's—is designed as a short, daily period of self-reflection and examination. Over a seven-day period, set aside some quiet time to ask yourself two specific questions each day:

Day 1: *What am I most grateful for today? And what am I least grateful for today?*

Day 2: *When did I give and receive the most love today? When did I give and receive the least love today?*

Day 3: *When did I feel most alive today? When did I feel the least alive today?*

Day 4: *What was the best thing that happened to me today? What was the worst thing that happened to me today?*

Day 5: *When did I have the greatest sense of belonging today? When did I have the least sense of belonging?*

Day 6: *When was I happiest today? When was I saddest today?*

Day 7: *What was today's high point? What was today's low point?*

As with the previous exercise, this one will help you to focus on what is happening around you. A busy lifestyle with many commitments rarely provides an opportunity for reflection and contemplation. Moments like these can bring insight and clarity that you can use in other areas of life, such as improving your awareness of triggers that create angry responses.

Don't Forget to Breathe

As simple as it sounds, paying attention to how we breathe can help us to feel better. When we live in a consistently angry emotional state, we tend to take short, shallow breaths from our chests to get more oxygen to our lungs quickly. Chest breathing is *stress breathing*. Do your own experiment and notice how you are breathing the next time you are upset about something.

EXERCISE 6.4 RELAXATION BREATHING

The preferred alternative to stress breathing is *relaxation breathing*. Start by breathing in through your nose, expanding your lungs and then exhaling through your mouth with a *whoosh*. As you practice this deep-breathing technique, exaggerate it so that you can feel the difference. With repetition, it will become more natural, and as an added benefit, you will become more aware of when your breathing pattern shifts into stress mode.

EXERCISE 6.5
FOUR-BY-FOUR-BY-FOUR BREATHING

Do this exercise at least three times a day and whenever else you have the opportunity. It is simple and easy, so practice it a lot! Using the previous deep-breathing technique, breathe *in* for four counts (through your nose and deep into your lungs), and breathe *out* for four counts (through your mouth with a *whoosh*) for around four minutes. This exercise will help you get a good supply of fresh oxygen into your lungs. It is refreshing and renewing, sort of like an adult time-out, and can help take the edge off your anger.

Make a Decision about Anger

No one can deny the fact that the challenges of being in a relationship with a partner who has ADHD can sometimes cause strong emotional reactions, and realistically, sometimes an angry response is entirely appropriate. You are entitled to have feelings and emotions, and it would be wrong to ignore or deny them. But if anger has become a way of life for you, if it has come to define who you are and how you are, then you are in a danger zone. A wise proverb states, "You will not be punished for your anger. You will be punished by your anger." Anger can destroy your quality of life, your satisfaction in relationships, and, most important, your physical and mental well-being. If you were sitting in front of me in a counseling session, I would speak very frankly and directly about your anger. I would tell you that a life filled with anger is an unhappy life and would encourage you to get to the source, to discover what is fueling the anger and to take the necessary steps to begin the healing process within yourself, regardless of your partner's ADHD behavior. It may take some work on your part, but by understanding the function of your anger, you will be able to move beyond it to a different way of life, one that is characterized by satisfaction, contentment, and fulfillment.

CHAPTER 7

Reality Check

There was a man who had been married for several years. Over time he noticed that whenever his wife prepared a ham for dinner, she always cut the end off the ham before she put it in the pan and cooked it. This seemed a little wasteful to the husband, so one day he asked, "Honey, when you cook a ham, why do you always cut the end off of it?" He thought perhaps it was a cooking technique, that maybe it helped seal the juices so that the ham would taste better or something like that. So he was surprised when she shrugged her shoulders and replied, "I do it because my mother always did it that way, and I figured that's the way it should be done." He then asked her if she had ever thought about not cutting the end off the ham when she cooked it. She looked at him for moment and asked, "Why would I do that?"

The next time his mother-in-law came to their house for dinner, he was reminded of his question to his wife about the ham, so he asked his mother-in-law if she was in the habit of cutting the end off a ham when she cooked it, and she responded affirmatively. When he asked her why, she answered, "I guess I thought that's the way it should be done because it's the way my mother always did it."

Now he was determined to get to the bottom of the mystery. Fortunately, Grandma was still living (and cooking), so the next day he and his wife called her and asked if, indeed, she always cut the end off a ham before cooking it, and she responded, "Yes, I do." Of course, they asked her why. Her response was, "I have an old stove with a small oven, so the only pan that fits is a small one. The ham is always too big to fit in the pan, so I have to cut the end off."

Grandma had a perfectly good reason for cooking the ham that way, but two more generations of women, who had modern appliances that could accommodate large hams, had mimicked her behavior for no good reason, except that they had thought it was the way a ham "should" be cooked. They had continued to cut the end off the ham without questioning it, because it had become the expected way to cook a ham.

Letting Go of the "Shoulds"

The ham story is a good illustration of how we become conditioned to have certain expectations: expectations about how things should be done, how life should be lived, and even what a relationship should be like. Both partners bring a set of expectations about how a relationship should be carried out, what each partner should do in the relationship. Just as there was an unspoken rule about how to cook a ham, we can have unspoken rules and assumptions about how to be in a relationship. Many times, no one questions any of these assumptions, even when it doesn't make sense to continue in the same way.

Many factors can contribute to "shoulds" in a relationship: *Ethnicity* can contribute in determining roles and responsibilities in a relationship. Certain cultures have very strong notions regarding the duties of men and women. Do you or your partner have any strong cultural influences that may be affecting your relationship? Even *birth order* can contribute to assumptions about what a role in a relationship is "supposed" to be: first-born males are expected to be leaders, middle children are expected to be compliant and get along with everyone, and the "baby" of the family is often allowed to escape responsibilities, sometimes even into adulthood.

Most important, *gender* can play a big part. What do you and your partner believe is the role of a woman in a relationship? What is the expected role of a man? Despite the fact that it's the twenty-first century, with few exceptions most relationships still rely on a traditional distribution of jobs and duties within the relationship. To some extent, the presumption is that a man should handle the finances, take care of household repairs, tend the yard, and manage the family automobiles. The same traditional relationship assumes that the woman keeps the house, shops for food and prepares it, takes care of the laundry, and manages the children's daily lives.

All of the assumptions that are carried into a relationship—whether they are passed down from generation to generation or based on gender, ethnicity, birth order, or traditional beliefs—can create a lot of "shoulds" that can adversely affect the relationship. When we have assumptions about responsibilities, we tend to project our expectations onto our partners. Many couples can fall captive to the "shoulds" when sorting out role expectations, but a couple with an ADHD partner is particularly vulnerable to falling into the "should" trap. The unsuspecting non-ADHD partner may be surprised when duties and responsibilities within the relationship aren't carried out in the way she expected. For instance, ADHD dynamics such as distractibility can lead to forgetfulness and lack of attention—even when important things are involved. And impulsivity can result in putting aside tasks to engage in other activities that are more interesting but don't necessarily serve the best interest of the relationship. The "shoulds," or the expected ways to do things in a relationship, may need to be reconsidered in a relationship involving a partner who has ADHD.

Renowned psychologist Albert Ellis often told his patients that they were "should-ing" all over themselves when they insisted on defining how things ought to be in life. Even though you are aware of ADHD symptoms and how they affect your partner, are you "should-ing" all over yourself? Is your ADHD partner forgetful? Then why do you expect him to remember all the time? Does he lack the attentiveness required to handle finances? Why do you carry resentment over this? Is your ADHD partner always late? Then what makes you think that he will be on time? Is he impulsive? Why do you continue to lose your temper and get upset when he plays golf instead of mowing the lawn?

The non-ADHD partner's expectations, if based on "shoulds," are usually too high and result in disappointment and dissatisfaction. This was the case with Rene. Despite being very familiar with the fact that her partner, Tom, had ADHD, she constantly complained, "Tom's a man, so he should do that." Rene had fallen into the "should" trap by continuing to hold on to unrealistic expectations of her partner with ADHD, largely based on her preconceived ideas about roles and responsibilities. Furthermore, Rene added another layer of "shoulds" by consistently comparing her relationship with Tom to their friends' relationships, often thinking things like *Doug would never do that in his relationship with Sally.* Everything seemed to contribute to Rene's dismay, leaving her feeling even more let down.

To help Rene put her complaints into proper perspective, I assigned a *stem completion exercise.* I instructed her to complete the following sentence with as many endings as she could think of:

My partner should be able to _____.

Rene came up with about twenty endings, and here are some samples:

My partner should be able to listen to and remember what I say.

My partner should be able to pay the bills on time.

My partner should be able to come home at a decent hour every evening.

Next, I asked Rene to examine each sentence within the context of Tom's ADHD to determine if the "should" statement was unreasonable and needed to be modified to meet the reality of his ADHD. Sheepishly, Rene admitted what she already knew was true: that all of her completed sentences needed some adjustment, particularly her insistence that Tom be home each night at the same time. As a result of going through the stem completion exercise, Rene carefully considered Tom's time management issues, along with the fact that he had a demanding job and a long commute. She now expects him to be late and makes her plans around that reality, rather than insisting that he be home at a certain time (and then getting annoyed when he isn't). Rene realized that it didn't make any sense to keep doing the same thing over and over again (being irritated when he was late), because the situation was not going to change (Tom was not going to become a punctual person). When Rene began to incorporate the impact of her husband's ADHD into her expectations, she found that she was better able to enjoy their time together no matter what time he arrived home.

Placing expectations on your ADHD partner that are too high or unrealistic contributes to your dissatisfaction, and the "shoulds" can get the best of you, as Rene discovered. The stem completion exercise is a constructive way to bring reality into your relationship. By becoming more realistic about your expectations, you may find that you can begin to experience more enjoyment in your relationship with your ADHD partner, rather than focus on your frustration and disappointment.

EXERCISE 7.1 STEM COMPLETION

1. Complete the following sentence with as many endings as you can think of: *My partner should be able to* _____ .

2. Examine each sentence within the context of your partner's ADHD to determine if the "should" statement is unreasonable.

3. Incorporate your new insight and understanding of the situation for the purpose of modifying your expectations.

Find Win-Win Solutions

David Neeleman, founder of JetBlue Airways, is a man who has come to terms with his ADHD and often speaks out about some of his challenges. He is up-front and honest about depending on others to take up the slack for him. In his discussions about ADHD (quoted in Gilman 2005), he indicates that he knows the value of surrounding himself with people who are good with the details of business. Your partner with ADHD may not be the CEO of a major corporation, but the stark reality is that any person with ADHD needs some help in managing life, sometimes on a daily basis. When you have a partner with ADHD, you are called on to facilitate, help out, and assist from time to time. Just keep in mind that helping out is different from taking on a responsibility. Helping out is using personal strengths and capacities to find solutions that work. Mr. Neeleman has found a win-win solution: he tackles the big picture and relies on the help of others to handle the details. Learning how to accommodate and work with your partner's ADHD can create win-win situations for everyone involved.

Janie's partner with ADHD was habitually late for work because of his difficulty with *activation*, which is the process of getting organized to do something. He had trouble waking up, getting dressed, and getting out the door on time. Rather than fussing, fuming, and complaining every day about her partner's tardiness, Janie set about to find ways to help him get more organized. For her, helping her partner with ADHD took the form of pointing things out and making suggestions; for example, Janie offered this idea: "Why don't we make sure that you put your watch and car keys right here every day so that you won't have to look for them every morning?" Her suggestion greatly helped her partner because he had not thought of putting his keys and watch in the same place each night. The outcome was that there was a little less disorganization and chaos in the house every morning, and they continued to work together to find solutions to other problems.

Another non-ADHD client, Jose, would call his wife every afternoon on his way home from work to see if there was anything she needed from the store. She frequently responded by saying, "Gee, I hadn't even thought of dinner yet." Jose knew that she had a tendency to get distracted during the day because of her ADHD and that time would get away from her. Rather than arrive home to find no dinner and no thoughts of dinner, and get upset about it, Jose purposefully made the call every day, not only in a sincere attempt to be helpful but also to help get her attention back on dinner preparations. Rather than complain about or criticize her for her time management problems, he found a positive way to help her manage the situation.

Maxine was very good at organizing her house and daily routines. She observed that her partner with ADHD, who was extremely creative, really enjoyed playing with their small son. They laughed and had marvelous, imaginative times together, and she realized that she didn't enjoy the playtime half as much as her partner seemed to. So she decided to use her gifts and talents of organization to make sure that each day was planned out and to set up all the essential details: food, activities, and schedules. Her partner with ADHD was free to care for their son using his artistic gifts and talents. For instance, she would be the one who made sure there was gas in the car so that they could all go to the park in the afternoon and have some fun. She let go of some of her expectations about her partner's responsibilities (in this instance, taking care of anything to do with the car) to capitalize on what he did bring to their relationship.

Florence found out early in her relationship with Lou, who had ADHD, that he was not great at saving or budgeting, and didn't even like discussing these issues. Even though she came from a family where her father had always managed the family finances, Florence, who was actually quite good with money matters, decided to take over the responsibility. Although sometimes she felt overwhelmed by all of her daily duties, she knew that she needed to take on the job of maintaining control of the family finances if they were to remain solvent. Even though paying the bills and keeping up with financial management used her valuable time, she decided that having control over this area gave her great peace of mind and was worth her effort. Florence was a smart woman who realized that it was better to assign roles based on competency and ability rather than expectations.

Finding win-win solutions is a healthy way to manage a relationship with a partner who has ADHD. Sometimes non-ADHD partners can't see the forest for the trees, and become too wrapped up in the "shoulds" that can obstruct full utilization of everyone's gifts and talents. The sooner you come to terms with the fact that the unusual struggles involved in ADHD require some sort of assistance from you, the easier it will be to step back, take a deep breath, and look for win-win solutions in your relationship. Find ways to celebrate your differences, and learn to work as a team. You will be much happier.

Beware of Making Attributions

Making an *attribution* is explaining someone else's behavior by assigning a cause or reason for it. We attribute the behavior that we observe to either external or internal causes. An *external attribution* explains behavior based on the current circumstance; in other words, something about the circumstances led to the behavior. And an *internal attribution* explains someone's behavior based on individual characteristics: internal attitudes, abilities, personality, or temperament. For example: instead of bringing her own lunch as she usually does, your friend is eating in the company cafeteria today. An internal attribution, which is personal, might be that she likes what is on the menu today. An external attribution, based on circumstances, could be that she left her lunch at home.

Here's the important part: We are more likely to attribute an internal, or personal, reason to a behavior when someone does something *that most people would not do* or when it is a behavior *that we don't understand.* For instance, if your friend tells you that he enjoys going to a lake house in the summer, you wouldn't think too much about his statement and wouldn't draw any conclusions about him, because it's not unusual for people to enjoy spending time at a lake in the summer. But if the same friend told you that he likes to go to Florida in the middle of hurricane season, you would look for an internal attribution to explain his behavior based on his interests or personality. You would make this internal attribution because you probably would not go to Florida during hurricane season and, in fact, most tourists stay away from Florida during hurricane season.

The tendency to assign an internal attribution to someone's behavior can create misunderstandings, because if we observe a behavior that we would not do or that most people would not do, we are inclined to make judgments about the person engaging in the behavior. And we tend to disregard other factors that can help to explain the behavior. ADHD behavior is wide open to internal attributions from others.

One young woman who had ADHD realized that her tendency to get distracted could cause her friends to make internal attributions about her behavior. She noticed that she had a hard time engaging in conversations, because the least little thing would distract her and she would look away to follow whatever had caught her interest: a random stranger walking by or a noise from the next room. She decided to ask one of her close friends if this was a problem. He told her that many times, he got the feeling that she wasn't interested in talking to him and that he often cut the conversation short because he thought she was being rude and he felt uncomfortable. The reason she had a hard time staying focused on conversations was her ADHD, not that she didn't care about her friend. But he didn't know it. Because most people maintain eye contact while having a conversation, he had attributed her behavior to an internal cause: that she was rude and somewhat self-centered. This was a wakeup call for the young woman, who began to fervently practice active listening skills, especially keeping eye contact throughout her conversations.

Now imagine your partner as he navigates a regular day. Which of his ADHD behaviors are others likely to mistakenly attribute to internal causes? Is he easily distracted by external stimuli, as the young woman was? Does he have trouble staying focused on conversations? Does he have trouble sitting still in meetings? Might his restlessness be sending a message that signals a lack of interest? Is his speech impulsive? Does he go off on tangents? Does he say things without processing the impact on others? Most people are able to keep eye contact in a conversation, most can sit still even in boring meetings, and most have a way of filtering their thoughts that keeps them from saying inappropriate things. Unless your partner wears a sign that says, "I have ADHD," chances are that he will be misunderstood often, and people around him will probably make a negative internal attribution about him.

It can be hard enough in the outside world, but unfortunately many non-ADHD partners also make internal attributions about the behaviors of their partners who have ADHD. A non-ADHD client said this: "One problem in our relationship is that my wife has a hard time listening and paying attention to me. It's difficult to try to maintain the idea that it's not because of me. I know it can be attributed to the ADHD, but I'm always tempted to feel insulted or slighted, or that I am uninteresting or unimportant." So many of the common complaints from non-ADHD partners are due to behaviors that are repeated over and over again in the relationship: not listening, not following through, procrastinating, and managing time poorly. The idea that most people who are in a committed relationship put forth the effort to listen to their partners, make sure a job gets done, and show up for important events makes it hard for the non-ADHD partner to have patience. Another of my non-ADHD clients puts it this way: "I frequently feel like I can't count on her, and I come away with a suspicion that she doesn't love me because she doesn't do what seem like simple things that she knows are important to me. And I know that if I knew something was important to her, I would go out of my way to make sure I did it."

Another non-ADHD client felt that her partner didn't really love her because he never seemed to remember their anniversary or her birthday. Despite her considerable knowledge of ADHD and its difficulties, there was still a part of her that felt that if he really cared, he would make sure he didn't forget. She said the only reason he remembered to buy her a Christmas present—which, by the way, was always done at the last possible minute—was that the whole world was aware of it and he couldn't escape the reminders. The reality was that her husband loved her very much and was personally devastated whenever he forgot an important date. Even though she had been married to her partner with ADHD for many years and was very familiar with the symptoms of the disorder, she confessed that in her "bad" moments, she still attributed her husband's behavior to internal causes and had to fight off feeling that he was uncaring, selfish, and too wrapped up in his own life to think of anyone else.

Be aware of and take care to guard against making too many internal attributions about your ADHD partner's behavior. Keep in mind that our natural tendency is to disregard other factors—even if we are fully aware of them—that can help to explain behavior. Remember to externalize the ADHD by reminding yourself every day of the following two things:

- Your partner has ADHD.

- Don't take it personally.

All Things Considered

Living with a partner with ADHD demands that you maintain a very realistic view of how ADHD can significantly affect your relationship. Take everything into consideration. Do you have any "shoulds" that need to be discarded for the good of the relationship? Are you still attempting to "cut the end off the ham" when it doesn't make any sense for you to do that anymore? Do you continue to attribute your partner's behavior to internal causes when you are fully aware of how ADHD can affect her behavior?

Take a few minutes to imagine how difficult it can be at times for your partner to try to manage his ADHD. Look for any effort that your partner makes to handle his ADHD. Appreciate any effort that you notice, and let him know. Keeping all of these things in mind will help ground you to the reality of living with a partner who has ADHD. Being grounded in reality will ultimately help you to live a life that is more fulfilling and enjoyable.

CHAPTER 8

Setting and Strengthening Personal Boundaries

Do you sometimes feel taken advantage of by your partner with ADHD and overburdened by your daily responsibilities? Do you have very little time left over for yourself? Do you feel as if you are the tour director who never gets to take a vacation? If so, it's probably safe to say that you might feel that your partner with ADHD ignores your personal boundaries from time to time. One woman shared with me that she feels as though her husband who has ADHD is driving a steamroller straight at her and that, more often than not, she feels flattened by the aftermath of his ADHD behavior.

What Are Personal Boundaries?

Generally, when we discuss our *personal boundaries*, we are referring to our emotional needs and preferences, and how they get played out in reciprocal interactions with everyone in our lives, especially our partners. *How do I like to be treated? What will I allow, and not allow, to be said and done to me? What seems appropriate to me, both verbally and physically? What are my priorities? What is my bottom line?* All of these questions can help define your personal boundaries. When your personal boundaries are strong, they provide you with a sense of protection and security. When your boundaries are poor or weak, you feel vulnerable and defenseless. One of my clients described boundaries in this way: "It's as though I've drawn an invisible circle around me. Inside my circle are my emotional, mental, and physical comfort levels. If someone tries to step inside my circle without an invitation, I feel threatened."

Understanding the notion of personal boundaries and being able to recognize them is an important factor in maintaining personal integrity. But sometimes people have trouble understanding the concept because they've grown up in families or lived in situations where personal boundaries were ignored, violated, or considered wrong or selfish. For instance, when a child isn't allowed to close the bathroom door, his personal boundary concerning privacy is not respected. A parent disclosing intimate information to a child breaches the child's personal boundary concerning appropriate interaction between a parent and a child. Or consider a little girl who feels appropriately sad about something but is told that she isn't allowed to be sad, that she has nothing to be sad about. Many adults who experienced these types of situations in childhood find it uncomfortable to have and express feelings concerning personal boundaries, or to expect their boundaries to be respected. It is never wrong or selfish to have emotional needs and preferences, and it is never wrong to express them, although we do need to take care to express them appropriately. Also, it is never wrong to reasonably expect your needs to be met and respected, especially by your partner.

Establishing and maintaining healthy boundaries for the purpose of developing emotional safety is at the core of implementing a healthy relational system. Feeling understood, appreciated, and respected by your partner allows you to relax and enjoy the relationship. When your personal boundaries are recognized and respected by others, especially those close to you, it's a great feeling. A sense of protection or emotional safety in the relationship is generated whenever you feel that your partner values your personal boundaries.

Usually, we don't go around every day thinking, *Here is my boundary* in this or that situation, but rather we become acutely aware of our boundaries when we feel that they have been violated, ignored, or disrespected. For example, Richard expressed to his stay-at-home wife who has ADHD that after a long day of commuting to and from, and working at, his stressful job, he would really appreciate it if he could come home to an orderly house. He told her nicely on several occasions why this was important to him: having the house in order would help him to feel calmer and more relaxed, and allow him to have more energy to be with his family. Having actually lowered his expectations over the years, he feels that his request is not extraordinary. The only time he expresses his displeasure is when he finds the kitchen sink piled full of dishes left over from the day before. That's when his frustration gets the best of him and he speaks to his wife in a heated manner. She usually responds in anger, the night is ruined, and nobody is happy. Richard feels that his wife consistently ignores or violates his personal boundary, a preference for an orderly house. The end result is that Richard feels unimportant to her and, more important, doesn't feel emotionally safe in the relationship.

When we feel that our personal boundaries have been violated or ignored, we instinctively feel a need to defend them. And in an effort to defend ourselves from feeling violated or ignored, we usually react in anger, as Richard did. If the violations become long-standing and remain unresolved, relational distress is the result. The distress creates conflict that tends to erupt quickly and then escalate. Consequently, tension resides in the home and everyone feels it. A lot of emotional wear and tear is created, on not only the relationship but also your personal sense of well-being. Many of my non-ADHD clients suffer from their own depression and anxiety, and also have various physical complaints: migraines, back problems, and digestive concerns. Quite often in counseling, once we begin the work of clarifying personal boundaries, the emotional and physical complaints begin to diminish.

A vital component of any healthy relationship is respecting each other's personal boundaries, but this can be problematic when you are in a relationship with someone with ADHD. Due to the symptoms associated with ADHD, the non-ADHD partner may feel that daily life comprises constant skirmishes to protect and defend personal boundaries. Here are some typical complaints:

- "When he says he will be home at six, he doesn't show up until seven or eight; he has a habit of losing track of time."

- "She tends to forget to recharge her cell phone, so I've learned that I can't depend on her if I need to get in touch with her."

- "I can't count on her for anything out of the ordinary. The day care center called me again yesterday; she forgot that she was supposed to pick up the kids, and I had to leave a meeting to pick them up."

- "I've put him on a cash-only basis; I got tired of his impulsive expenditures, which drained our bank account."

While these examples can seem insignificant when compared to the larger issues in life, over time they can add up and feel overwhelming. The expectation of having personal boundaries respected and acknowledged can fade away due to the problematic behaviors and unfulfilling communication patterns associated with ADHD. Out of frustration, the non-ADHD partner gets angry and resentful. Anger and resentment can lead to discouragement, and many non-ADHD partners give up, feeling defeated, and discontinue any attempts to get their personal boundaries recognized and respected. A common attitude is "What's the use? It doesn't seem to make a difference." If you feel angry and discouraged, maybe you've given up and lost hope of having your partner value your boundaries. Let me be a voice in the wilderness that says, "Don't give up! Hang in there! It's worth fighting for!" You and your partner with ADHD may have fallen into unfulfilling, unsatisfactory habits and patterns of interaction. Your partner with ADHD has many good qualities that attracted you in the first place, but you've probably lost sight of them over time due to the problems created by ADHD symptoms. It's worth a renewed effort to establish and learn how to defend your personal boundaries so that you can rediscover relational satisfaction.

Beginning the Journey of Establishing Personal Boundaries

We have already established that it's okay to have personal boundaries and that you deserve to have your partner recognize and respect them.

Next comes the hard part: you need to get comfortable with being more assertive in stating your boundaries and communicating your feelings when your boundaries feel violated. Don't mistake assertive for aggressive. While both attitudes express wants, needs, and feelings, aggressiveness means acting in an antagonistic manner, using angry words and gestures. Aggressive behavior may get us what we want in the short term but is ultimately detrimental to a relationship. Assertive behavior is more controlled and is delivered with confidence; there is no need for angry words and gestures.

Learning how to express your needs and desires assertively will significantly contribute to your emotional and physical health. You will experience more peace and personal contentment, and much less stress. While the concept is simple, it may not be easy. Realistically, creating and preserving our personal boundaries with a partner who has ADHD doesn't happen overnight. It takes a fair amount of thinking, planning, and consistent practice. I can't promise that it will be a comfortable process or that your partner who has ADHD will immediately respond in a positive manner, but I do believe it is worth it. The process begins with a couple of very important exercises, which will help put you in touch with hopes and expectations that you may have felt were forever lost. The result is that you will be able to express your desires, needs, and feelings with more clarity and less emotion. You will have a healthier plan for effecting change in your relational life.

EXERCISE 8.1 TAKING INVENTORY

The first step in creating healthy personal boundaries is to take a personal inventory of your life. Find a quiet time and place, where you can devote some uninterrupted energy to examining what is going on in your daily relationship with your partner who has ADHD. Have some paper, a notebook or journal, or your laptop computer handy for writing down your thoughts. After you are comfortable and centered, begin to ask yourself the following questions:

- *What makes me feel content, in my own life and in my life with others?*

- *What makes me feel productive and effective?*

- *When have I felt most content, productive, and effective? What was going on then? What has changed?*

- *What gets in the way of my feeling content, productive, and effective?*

- *How have I tried to change the things that get in the way?*

- *Have those efforts worked?*

- *If not, is there anything that I could do differently in the future?*

You probably won't be able to finish the exercise in one sitting and, in fact, may feel overwhelmed once you begin. If you are like most non-ADHD partners, this may be the first time in a long time, or perhaps the first time ever, that you have allowed yourself to wonder about these highly emotional issues. So you may experience a lot of feelings while doing this exercise, and that might make it hard at first. You may feel very sad over lost opportunities, or perhaps long-buried feelings of anger might surface. Consider this a normal consequence of the exercise. Taking some extra time to write about these emerging feelings will be beneficial in the long run. (It's important to note here that if you are having difficulty figuring out what healthy boundaries would be for you, then seek help from a counselor or therapist, especially one who understands ADHD.)

The inventory exercise involves time and thought. Don't give up or become distressed by the emotions; come back and continue to work on the exercise. Be patient with yourself; you are beginning the process of getting a clearer picture of who you are and what you need. More than likely, your personal needs, wishes, desires, and priorities may have taken a backseat to the demands brought about by living with someone who has ADHD, so it may take some time for clarity to emerge.

EXERCISE 8.2 WHAT YOU WON'T DO ANYMORE AND WILL DO IN THE FUTURE

Your personal inventory exercise helped you to take a serious look at yourself, your life, and your circumstances. This next exercise is an important one, because now you will need to decide what you won't do anymore and what you will do instead. You will be replacing old, dysfunctional ways of expressing your desires and needs with ones that are healthier by creating a "won't do / will do" list.

Once again, get some paper, a notebook, your journal, or a laptop computer, and find some time to be alone and uninterrupted. Make three columns on your paper. Label the leftmost column "Problem," and list there the relational patterns that seem to be problematic and ongoing with your partner who has ADHD. Be sure to take the time to list *all* the issues you can think of, because each problematic situation will need a separate response. Here's a word of caution: you may hesitate to finish this exercise because you might perceive it as too negative, too problem focused. Once you write down all of the problems and see them in black and white, you may feel overwhelmed and want to give up. Don't despair; this exercise is all about change, so creating a realistic and thorough problem list is absolutely vital for you to come up with different ways of handling your emotional, verbal, and physical reactions to your partner with ADHD in order to create better personal boundaries.

Next, as you think about each problem on your list, consider what maladaptive responses to each problem you have made in the past. Getting angry, nagging, or giving the silent treatment are common responses. Put the responses that you have used in the past but want to change in the middle column, titled "What I Won't Do Anymore." For instance, after reflection, you may realize that you usually respond with a sarcastic comment when you feel disappointed about something your partner with ADHD has or hasn't done. You've realized that you don't like to respond sarcastically, that it doesn't feel good, so you write "Respond sarcastically" in this column.

Now that you have identified the problems in your relationship that tend to cause you aggravation and your own patterns of unsuccessful and unrewarding responses, the next step is to consider what would be a better response when the problem arises again (and it will). Make a third column on your paper with the heading "What I Will Do in the Future." In this column, write down your new, healthier, and more adaptive reactions to the same situation. The important thing to do here is to come up with a response or action that is more reasoned and less emotionally driven.

I once counseled a woman named Marie, who was married to Dave, who had ADHD, combined type. She was at her wit's end, complaining of a constant state of irritation with Dave. Anger wasn't Marie's main emotion anymore; she complained of being tired of her relationship, declaring that she was worn out and "done." Her anger at not having her boundaries respected in her marriage had morphed into despair about the future. I worked with Marie to help her rediscover her long-buried personal boundaries. She was resistant at first because she felt that it wouldn't do any good and believed she would actually feel worse. But with a lot of encouragement, she completed her inventory and then tackled the "won't do / will do" list with renewed energy. Following is an example of two problems from Marie's list:

Problem	What I Won't Do Anymore	What I Will Do in the Future
Dave avoids conversations about money.	Badger and nag him. Get angry at his avoidance.	Have more awareness of the appropriate time to approach him. Ask permission to have the conversation. If he avoids the conversation, voice my frustration in a calm manner. If necessary, make money decisions on my own.
Dave forgets and messes up, and then tries to blame me.	Respond defensively. Lecture him about screwing up again.	Listen calmly. Offer empathy. Let him experience the consequences of his actions. Leave the room if he continues blaming me.

Marie's partial list (she had other problems to work through) is a good example of her attempts to generate new patterns of reaction to her partner who had ADHD. She wanted to change her angry and defensive responses to ones that were calmer and more evenhanded. Although Marie's relationship with Dave remained challenging, she began to feel much better about herself as she used her "won't do / will do" list to guide her. She also discovered that her worn-out feeling was actually a low level of depression, which began to lift after she started paying more attention to her own needs and desires in the relationship and when she began to communicate them in a different manner.

If you go through this process solely to get your ADHD partner to change, you will be disappointed. Your main objective in creating a "won't do / will do" list is to bring about a change in the way *you* behave, the way you conduct yourself. Your attempts to change are for your benefit. Any corresponding change in your partner who has ADHD will come about only if you change your behavior, your responses, and your reactions. Over time, as you cease reacting in a negative way and manage your responses in a healthier manner, there will be fewer opportunities for your partner to interact with you in the same old way. The emphasis will shift from your anger or irritation at your partner to the real issue: the ADHD-fueled behavior.

The "won't do / will do" list also helps you to create realistic goals for future action. Having a goal in mind helps you to make decisions on a daily basis.

• Carolina

Another client, Carolina, created a "won't do / will do" list that included what she wouldn't do and what she would do differently when her ADHD husband Jacob's latest project became abandoned and unattended due to his lost interest. Rather than think (or hope) that it wouldn't happen again and then get very upset when it did, this way she crafted a plan for the future. She reported that she felt better immediately just because she felt mentally and emotionally prepared.

Soon enough she had a situation that enabled her to put her plan into action. Her problem list had included the following:

"Jacob leaves things undone." She came home one afternoon to discover her husband's latest home improvement project left unfinished all over the garage floor. Jacob's leaving his project unfinished was bothersome enough for Carolina, because she knew that it would likely remain unfinished for a long time, but this particular unfinished project prevented her from parking her car in the garage, which increased her irritation. Carolina didn't like to complain and nag, which was why she had already written "Nagging and complaining to him to clean up his mess" in her "What I Won't Do Anymore" column. She had also completed her "What I Will Do in the Future" column in preparation for this exact circumstance.

Here was her plan: she would ask him, calmly but firmly, once a day for three days, if he had a time frame for either completing his project or cleaning it up. She felt that this would give him a reasonable amount of time to respond, and she was comfortable with waiting for up to three days. If there was no response or action (that is, the stuff wasn't cleaned up and put away) after the third request, then she would tell him again, calmly and firmly, that she was going to put the things away herself. Every day, she had a plan that governed her behavior and helped her to contain her feelings, and this felt really good to her. She reported that although she felt annoyed that she had to clean up his mess, she wasn't overcome or eaten up by anger or resentment as she might have been in the past. Consequently, her general mood was less irritated, and she had more emotional and mental energy to focus on other things. Carolina found the "won't do / will do" list very empowering.

Regardless of the frustrations that are encountered with a partner who has ADHD, you are the only one responsible for how you respond, and there is usually a better, more measured reaction in you somewhere, if you take some time to think about it and plan for it. You've probably spent many years putting up with troublesome behaviors from your partner with ADHD and may have run out of patience. You need to reset, reboot, and make positive, healthy changes in your life.

Ready, Set, Go: Putting Your Plan into Action

When you have taken an inventory of your personal boundaries based on your needs and desires, and made some decisions as to what you won't do anymore and what you will do in the future, you are ready to put your plan into action.

Now you are better equipped to communicate with your partner with ADHD when items on your problem list arise. For a more positive outcome, there are a few things to remember. First, when you communicate with your partner who has ADHD, it's important to choose an optimal time. Try not to have this talk during a football game, in the middle of an interesting movie, or the moment your partner walks through the front door. It's better to make sure, as best you can, that you choose a favorable time. You might want to have the talk in the morning, because the ADHD brain seems to be able to focus better in the morning, or try to do it after a meal. Perhaps a walk together in the evening would present an opportune moment. By choosing a more favorable time, you increase your odds of obtaining a positive outcome. *When* you communicate can be almost as important as *how* you communicate, especially with partners who have ADHD, because there are so many things that impede their ability to pay attention: the telephone rings or a text message comes in, the television is on, or the kids are running in and out. Finding a time when distractions are fewer will enhance the outcome.

Next, it's important to communicate in a manner that demonstrates how much you care so that you don't come across as complaining or criticizing. To do this, there are two components to keep in mind. First, ask permission to speak about your concerns. This approach conveys courtesy and respect to your partner. So you might say something like this: "Hey, honey, I've got some things on my mind, and I'm wondering if it would be okay to share them with you," or "I've been thinking about some things lately and would like discuss them with you." Chances are your partner will say, "Sure, what's up?" You will have better opportunities to bring up issues that might ordinarily be avoided or denied when you ask for and receive permission.

Second, during the conversation, it's important to use "I" statements to express your feelings. Please don't start by saying, "Your doing this or that is driving me crazy, and I can't stand it anymore, so let me tell you what is going to happen." Those are *finger-jabbing* (imagine jabbing your index finger in your partner's face) comments that will most likely elicit a very defensive response, defeating the purpose of the conversation. The "I" statement formula goes like this: "When I _____, I feel _____, and I would prefer _____." To demonstrate this approach, let's look at Leo and Jane, a couple who were having some trouble in their relationship.

• Leo and Jane

As working parents, Leo and Jane shared many of the housekeeping and child-rearing responsibilities. In fact, Leo was the cook in the family and enjoyed preparing meals for Jane and their children. But Jane, who was the ADHD partner, had an impulsive habit of bringing home coworkers or clients for dinner without letting Leo know in advance.

This bothered Leo, who noticed that this predicament seemed to crowd his thoughts more and more, so he wrote it in the "Problem" column on his "won't do / will do" list. He had discovered that he was behaving a little edgier than usual, especially around dinnertime, when he anticipated the possibility of surprise guests. His usual easygoing demeanor was becoming more negative, and he didn't like what was happening to him. His responses to Jane had become more clipped. He noticed that he was quieter than usual and less likely to join in dinnertime conversation. On reflection, he realized that he had hoped these cues would have communicated his annoyance to Jane and that she would have responded, but they didn't. Rather than simmer and stew, Leo came up with an idea for what he would do: he would talk to Jane about the problem.

Leo decided to bring up the subject to Jane one evening while they were taking a walk after dinner. He chose that time because there was no hunger to cause distraction, and they were alone, without any household interruptions. He had her full attention, an important factor with a partner who has ADHD. At an appropriate moment, he asked her if he could share something that was on his mind. Her response was positive; she said, "Yes, of course."

Leo had practiced what he was going to say and made sure to use "I" statements. He said, "Jane, honey, you know, when I have to accommodate extra people for dinner without any advance notice, I feel kind of disregarded and unimportant, and it would be better for me if you would give me at least a half day's notice. That way I could be prepared and would enjoy our guests more." Jane was very responsive; she'd had no idea that her impulsive hospitality was causing any problems for her husband. It would have been a different outcome had Leo told Jane that he was sick and tired of her inconsiderate behavior and wasn't going to put up with it anymore.

After you have had the talk, during which you have asked permission to voice your concerns and used effective "I" statements to communicate your concerns, then follow up your conversation with a concise e-mail or text message to your ADHD partner that summarizes what you discussed. E-mails and text messages are great ways to convey information; they are quick, easy, and convenient. But more important, they provide protection against the common ADHD complaint "You never told me" or "I didn't know I was supposed to." If you can't use text messages or e-mails, then write out a concise summary of your conversation on brightly colored paper or sticky notes. (I recommend neon orange, yellow, pink, or green. The bright colors are better for grabbing the attention of the partner who has ADHD.) Leo wrote an e-mail to Jane the next day that said, "Hey honey, I really enjoyed our walk last night. Thank you so much for keeping me in mind before you invite guests for dinner." His message was perfect: quick, concise, and clear.

There's one other thing to note: keep your options open for possible changes in the future. Despite your best efforts at thinking through certain situations, things may not work as planned, or your circumstances may change. Or you may find that your expectations concerning personal boundaries are unreasonably high. Life and its issues are not static, but are ever changing, so it is perfectly permissible to make different decisions in the future.

Personal boundaries are as essential to our emotional health as food, air, and water are to our physical health. Because they are so vital, it is worth all of the time, energy, and effort that are required to make them healthy and strong. If your partner with ADHD has been inattentive to your personal boundaries in the past, you may feel that it is too late to do anything about it. An old Chinese proverb says that the best time to plant a tree was thirty years ago, but the next best time to plant a tree is today. Intend to start today to build personal boundaries that will lead you toward health, satisfaction, and contentment.

Remember that understanding and communicating our boundaries, which include feelings, desires, and needs, is critical to creating personal and relational health. If your partner breaches your boundaries, anger and resentment are likely to surface, so it is important to examine and change ineffective patterns. Conveying a kind but firm resolve that demonstrates consistency is the best strategy for change.

CHAPTER 9

Recognizing and Avoiding Relational Roadblocks

On occasion, even the most successful relationships fail to be satisfying and fulfilling, due to the stressors brought on by life issues and circumstances. When life stressors show up, *relational roadblocks*—defined as anything that prohibits a relationship from being mutually satisfying and fulfilling—can arise. When relational roadblocks arise, couples may find that their communication falters and their ability to resolve conflict breaks down. When the symptoms of ADHD are added to the challenges brought on by life stressors, the potential for even more relational roadblocks increases, at times to the point of seeming insurmountable.

It's hard to be in a relationship where you feel as though you must constantly pick up the pieces left strewn about by your partner with ADHD, so it's easy to put the blame on ADHD symptoms for creating relational roadblocks: "If only my partner would listen to me when I talk to him, I wouldn't have to keep reminding him and nagging him, which he hates," or "If only my partner would learn to finish what she starts, I wouldn't need to keep after her and wouldn't get so mad." Dynamics prompted by ADHD symptoms are problematic and do cause relational distress, but very little is ever mentioned about how the non-ADHD partner may also be contributing to relational roadblocks. I have found that, when used in an unhealthy way, some of the innate capabilities and strengths that the non-ADHD partner brings to the relationship (such as organization, thoroughness, stability, and punctuality) can actually become part of the problem.

In this chapter we will examine three common and problematic relational roadblocks that can unintentionally and inadvertently be brought on by a non-ADHD partner's capabilities and strengths. And we will investigate opportunities for avoiding the roadblocks in the future so that your relationship can move toward becoming a more successful, mutually satisfying partnership.

Roadblock One: Overhelping and Excessive Caretaking

It is not unusual for a person with ADHD to seek out and be attracted to a partner who will bring steadiness and constancy to the relationship (Betchen 2003). Taking this into consideration, you are probably competent in the following areas: organization, time management, follow-through, and impulse control. You are most likely a person who is capable and helpful. You might consider yourself strategic: you can take control of a situation and create order out of chaos, figuring out what needs to be done in most situations and then doing it. You are the go-to person when things need to get done. Also, you are probably reliable and punctual. Others know that when you commit to something, you will follow through; you can be counted on. You are also likely to be pretty good at taking care of others, even anticipating their needs before they do on most occasions. Empathy and authentic concern for others may be a natural quality in you; that's why you are good at helping. In addition to these skills, you also might be considered emotionally stable, less likely to blow up in anger or frustration. All of these characteristics create a pretty impressive skill set, and the people whom you are close to are fortunate to have you around. You are a valuable asset, especially to a partner with ADHD, because you are able to put things back in order when life gets messy.

Overhelping

All of your well-intentioned, useful strengths that are meant to benefit the relationship can also create situations in which you *overhelp*. Despite your good intentions, overhelping can contribute to relational difficulties. Consider these scenarios:

- Overhelping, or taking up too much slack for your partner with ADHD, can result in enabling, and a state of unhealthy dependency can develop.

- Over time you may begin to anticipate future situations and step in (or interfere) before your partner with ADHD needs help.

- Your partner with ADHD may come to resent you for overhelping.

- By overhelping, you can get physically run down and emotionally and mentally worn out, and might give up completely, resulting in a "Who cares?" attitude.

- Destructive communication patterns can develop as a consequence of overhelping.

Most partners with ADHD benefit from assistance from their non-ADHD partner and often rely on the non-ADHD partner to step in, to fill in the gaps when problems arise. But if the goal in a healthy relationship is to be equal partners, the tendency to overhelp can cause relational imbalance, creating a roadblock to mutual satisfaction and fulfillment in the relationship.

Excessive Caretaking

Overhelping is detrimental to a relationship, but some non-ADHD partners take it to an extreme, resulting in *excessive caretaking*. Excessive caretaking occurs when you become too absorbed, too wrapped up—almost to an obsessive degree—in managing your ADHD partner's life. This type of caretaking can result in a relational roadblock that includes some extremely unhealthy relational dynamics. Constantly checking up on your ADHD partner (I'm not talking about "checking in"; that's different) many times during the day to see if he has completed tasks; running interference with family, neighbors, friends, or bosses to keep your partner from doing or saying anything that could cause trouble; or staying up until the wee hours of the morning (while your partner sleeps) to finish paperwork that he needs the next day for a work deadline are a few examples of excessive caretaking.

A certain degree of sacrificing personal wants and needs is required in intimate relationships. Ideally, relationships are reciprocal, following the rule "I'll look after you, and you'll look after me." Concern equals caring. When you care about your partner's welfare, you consider the following: *What is going on with my partner? What might she need? Can I meet that need without surrendering too much of myself?* While an appropriate amount of sacrifice can be a necessary dynamic in a relationship because it shows concern, excessive caretaking takes sacrifice to an unhealthy level. Getting wrapped up in an excessive caretaking cycle means being too involved in another's life, so much so that it affects the relationship and each partner's quality of life. Furthermore, overinvolvement in another's life requires putting your own needs at a much lower priority, creating imbalance.

Let's take a look at some of the characteristics of a non-ADHD partner who might be an excessive caretaker:

- *I worry about what my partner with ADHD will do or say when I'm not around.*

- *I feel responsible for the actions of my partner who has ADHD.*

- *I do more than my share of everything.*

- *I must exert control by constantly checking up on my partner who has ADHD.*

- *I feel persistently edgy and nervous even when there is nothing to be concerned about.*

- *I have difficulty with asserting myself and expressing my feelings to my partner who has ADHD.*

- *I have trouble asking for help.*

- *I feel helpless to effect change in my life.*

- *I never take time for myself.*

If any of these descriptors feels familiar, ask yourself these questions (writing out your responses could help you gain insight):

- *Why do I feel this way, and why do I do what I do? (Am I fearful of what might happen if I step back? Am I disappointed about how my relationship has turned out? Have I given up any expectations for change?)*

- *Am I doing anything to make it worse? (How have I participated? What is my responsibility?)*

- *What do I need to change? (Am I willing to make changes for the sake of my relationship? Even if it is difficult?)*

If you recognize a tendency in yourself toward excessive caretaking, it's important to pay attention to how you might be actively participating and to think of new ways to approach your relational situations. Some of your solutions will involve making different decisions about how you think or act.

• George and His Partner with ADHD

George realized that he was an excessive caretaker to his ADHD partner when he noticed that whenever his partner had to travel, he would go into a tizzy trying to make sure she was ready and off in time so that she wouldn't miss her flight. He felt responsible for her and also felt that if he didn't try to control her, she would fail. While his partner went to bed and got a good night's sleep, George would stay up late the night before the trip, packing her suitcase and making sure that she had everything. Then he got up early the next day for the purpose of reminding her every few minutes to keep on task. George put all of his own responsibilities on hold so that he could successfully get his partner out the door on time. When she finally left for the airport, George would almost collapse out of nervous exhaustion, and it took him most of the day to recover.

He realized that, over time, he had become an active contributor to this unhealthy pattern and was not happy with himself. To "unhook" from excessive caretaking, George felt that he needed to stop trying to control his partner. After asking himself the three questions previously listed, George realized that making the flight was more important to him than to his partner, so he decided that he would let her figure things out in the future, even if that meant missing a flight. Using this as a template, he was able to unhook from similar situations, and said he had more peace in his life than he had experienced in a long time.

• Louise and Her Partner with ADHD

Another client, Louise, identified with many of the items on the excessive caretaking list but especially the last one: "I never take time for myself." She shared with me that she had been a competitive swimmer when she was younger and had almost forgotten how much she loved to swim. Out of genuine care and concern, she had become overinvolved in micromanaging the life of her partner with ADHD, which left her very little time to do anything for herself, including swimming. The sadness brought on by remembering how she used to feel in the pool almost overwhelmed her. But rather than feel sorry for herself, she was motivated into action.

The very next day, she went to her local Y and signed up for a membership, and now she swims at least three times a week, sometimes more. Louise gave herself permission to take care of herself and, as a result, feels much better. She also reported that when she began to practice good self-care, she found it easier to begin the process of letting go of her need to control other areas of her partner's life. Taking good care of yourself by adding pleasurable events, such as exercising, may seem like an insignificant step in tackling the bigger issues, such as control and worry, but it can open up new ways of feeling and thinking that naturally lead to making other good decisions that can have a positive effect on your relational life.

Overhelping and excessive caretaking occur when you take too much responsibility for your partner who has ADHD. Consider this rhetorical question: If your partner is cold, why are you putting on a coat? This means that if you are taking too much ownership of your partner's ADHD-related problems and trying to put your solutions in place, then you aren't allowing your partner a chance to figure things out for himself and learn how to take care of his own needs. Louise and George were always micromanaging their partners' lives and consistently rescuing them from the consequences of their actions. Once they decided to let their partners put on their own "coats," so to speak, their relationships began to improve.

When Louise realized that she took on too many life responsibilities that belonged to her partner, she was able to pull back (not pull away; she still offered to help). George reported that he was more likely to wait for his partner to ask for assistance, rather than bulldoze ahead of her. Both Louise and George came to understand that finding a better balance ultimately made them into better partners who were more effective at giving the appropriate amount of help and assistance when it was needed.

Roadblock Two: Learned Helplessness

Overhelping and excessively caretaking for your partner with ADHD can create a form of learned helplessness. *Learned helplessness* refers to a person's conditioned belief that she isn't capable of doing anything or accomplishing anything. For example, parents' insistence on doing their child's homework instead of allowing the child to do her own work and learn from the experience creates the groundwork for learned helplessness. At some point, if Mom and Dad aren't around for some reason, the child is faced with having to do her own work. But because she has never been allowed to take on the task of homework on her own, she has come to believe that she is incapable of doing homework. Furthermore, because she believes that she is incapable, she won't even try. She has learned how to be helpless.

Because the non-ADHD partner is usually better and faster at managing the details of everyday life—shopping, cooking, cleaning, planning, managing finances, and so on—there is a tendency for her to take on all of these jobs. Over time, this naturally diminishes the ADHD partner's responsibilities in the relationship. The non-ADHD partner eventually feels overburdened and, out of frustration, complains, "Why can't you help me? Why don't *you* do anything?" The partner who has ADHD is surprised because, over the course of the relationship, he has received a clear message that he can't do anything or that he can't do it as well, as fast, or as thoroughly as the non-ADHD partner. As a result, the partner with ADHD feels incapable of accomplishing or achieving very much and, like the child in the homework situation, doesn't even try.

• Belinda and Nathan

Belinda's predisposition to take on too many responsibilities in her relationship with Nathan, who had ADHD, caused her to overdo. He complained for a time because he truly wanted to participate in the relationship. But after a while he stopped complaining and kind of "gave up," as he said. When their tenth wedding anniversary came about and he didn't plan anything special for them, Belinda was appalled. Nathan's response was chilling: "You tell me that you always have to do everything because I never do anything right, so why would I even try?" Belinda had helped to create Nathan's learned helplessness. Her belief that she was using her abilities to help him out made it difficult for her to understand how this was contributing to Nathan's lack of responsibility. It took a lot of work for them to slowly deconstruct this unhealthy dynamic in their relationship.

EXERCISE 9.1 ARE YOU SETTING YOUR PARTNER UP FOR LEARNED HELPLESSNESS?

Are you in danger of feeding or initiating learned helplessness in your partner with ADHD? Do you find it easier to do things yourself, because your partner with ADHD doesn't do them fast enough or thoroughly? Here's a way to evaluate your situation:

1. On a piece of paper, list all of your responsibilities (other than job related) that have to be carried out on a day-to-day and week-to-week basis.

2. On a separate piece of paper, list all of your ADHD partner's responsibilities (other than job related) that must be carried out on a day-to-day and week-to-week basis.

3. Compare your list of responsibilities with your partner's and notice whether you have too many. If so, consider which tasks could be transferred out of your domain and into your partner's.

Belinda discovered that her list of responsibilities was out of proportion to Nathan's. She realized that she had taken over many responsibilities that Nathan was very capable of handling. The previous exercise was her first step in figuring out how to make adjustments for the purpose of bringing more balance back into the relationship and improving Nathan's sense of his own capability. It was hard at first because Nathan's inattentive-type ADHD often meant that he was slower in taking on responsibilities and slower with follow-through. It required that Belinda increase her patience with him and allow him to move at his own pace. With honesty and a lot of effort, they were able to create a much healthier and more enjoyable marriage.

Roadblock Three: The Parent Trap

Communication is vital in a relationship, because it's how we transmit information to each other. One way that we communicate is verbally, through the words that we use. Partners experiencing conflict might find themselves engaging in angry, sarcastic, and harsh communication. But in addition to words, a large part of what we communicate to each other is through nonverbal communication: facial expressions, posture, and other body language. Nonverbal messages can speak loud and clear, conveying anger, irritation, and discontent. In my counseling office, I pay special attention to a couple's nonverbal cues: Are his arms crossed over his chest? Maybe he's feeling defensive or hostile. If she rolls her eyes when he speaks, she's giving a pretty good clue to her negative emotional state.

If you overhelp or excessively caretake, causing your ADHD partner to feel incompetent, helpless, and overdependent, you are both likely to succumb to unhealthy patterns of communication, both verbal and nonverbal. A relationship involving ADHD is particularly vulnerable to a communication roadblock that I call the *parent trap*, in which the non-ADHD partner approaches and relates to the partner with ADHD as a parent would treat a disobedient child, by speaking in a harsh, punitive, parental manner. Left alone, unrecognized and unchanged, the parent trap can be so toxic that the end result is that the couple either splits up or stays together in misery (which affects everyone around them). But there is another alternative: if you learn to identify this pattern and realize when you are participating in it, you can resist falling into the parent trap, and the relationship will have a better chance of becoming more satisfying and fulfilling.

To illustrate, let's say a non-ADHD partner with organizational and time management skills has taken on the responsibility of making sure her time-challenged ADHD partner gets up, out of the house, and off to work on time. What might that scenario look like? She may begin to communicate her concern at first by saying, "Honey, you'd better hurry up; you are going to be late again." As time passes and the partner with ADHD seems no closer to being ready to leave, the non-ADHD partner might notch up the communication a bit and try to coax him with a reward or trickery (such as setting the clocks in the house forward fifteen minutes). If that doesn't work, she probably begins to nag, saying something like, "You're not ready *yet*? I can't believe it! What is taking you so long?" or maybe she nags nonverbally, with a big sigh, a shake of her head, or a pained facial expression.

The next level is exasperation, so the comments may become personal commentaries, such as "When are you ever going to learn how to be responsible and take care of yourself?" or "I can't believe how irresponsible you are; when will you ever learn?" While she has resorted to these methods to try to get her partner out of the house and on his way to work, as these communications escalate they become less effective at achieving that goal. Yet her frustration may swallow her up so that she begins delivering even more powerful reminders, with a sterner and more severe tone of voice: "If you don't hurry up and leave, you are going to be in big trouble, Mister." And sadly, she might resort to even harsher attempts, such as expressing her intense anger through yelling and name-calling.

What does her partner with ADHD do in response? He usually stays quiet at first and ignores her, maybe mumbles a comment or two under his breath. But before very long, his frustration kicks in, his anger escalates, and he begins to respond by yelling, "Leave me alone, will you!" "Stop telling me what to do!" or "I am not a child; stop treating me like one!" Finally, he gets fed up and stomps out of the house in anger. Both are glad to be away from each other.

This couple is firmly enmeshed and caught up in the parent trap. This dynamic throws the couple into a relational downward spiral, because when the partner with ADHD is spoken to or treated like child, he is more than likely to respond by acting like a child: picture a kid with his hand on his hip, looking defiantly at his parent and saying, "You're not the boss of me!" Playing out this dynamic day after day, week after week, and year after year can result in deep-seated resentment and bitterness in both partners. All other communication goes down the toilet, and the couple can barely say, "Pass the salt," to each other.

The partner who has ADHD complains of feeling constantly scolded and admonished, and tires of being told over and over again what to do and how to do it. The non-ADHD partner complains, "I've already asked nicely five or six times, but there is no response and I feel ignored. Yelling at him is the only way to get his attention." The frustration level grows, the intensity increases, and then the non-ADHD partner resorts to doing whatever needs to be done—even yelling and name-calling—to get the partner with ADHD to complete the task at hand. That's when the words and feelings escalate, as they did for the couple in the example. They were weary and frustrated from the all-too-familiar pattern, and neither knew how to get untangled from it.

If you find that you can relate—at any level—to what was just described, then be *very* careful about how you communicate your wants and needs to your partner. You are in great danger of falling into the parent trap and coming across as a nagging, complaining, punitive parent. Along with your words, your tone of voice, body language, and facial expressions communicate volumes. Remember that speaking to someone as though he were a child will probably elicit a childish response.

As if angry words and hurt feelings weren't enough, there are other consequences to the parent trap. As our behavior becomes more entrenched—that is, the more childish one partner acts, the more parental the other partner feels compelled to be, and vice versa—the original reason why the conflict erupted gets lost. Whatever caused the parent-child interaction to start in the first place is now forced to take a backseat to the angry words and hurt feelings. The spotlight becomes focused on how a partner was spoken to rather than on the original problem, and consequently, you are now several times removed from resolving the issue at hand. Any opportunity for understanding and potential for change are lost. No matter how frustrated you become, speaking the way a parent would speak to a disobedient child will not get you what you want in the long run. It may create enough stimulation to get your partner with ADHD moving, but if a healthy, mutually satisfying relationship is your goal, this is not the way to get it. It's important to learn how to disengage from this in order to keep from falling into the parent trap.

Another significant hazard of the parent trap is the deterioration of sexual intimacy in the relationship. Sex is best experienced when each partner feels respected and well regarded by the other. When the parent trap is alive and well, neither partner feels inclined toward sex, because the communication dynamic removes feelings of respect and consideration. One male client with ADHD told me that after week upon week of feeling as if he were living with his mother (because of the way his partner treated him), he had a hard time switching back to feeling like a sexual partner when he got into bed at night. Non-ADHD partners, observing their partners' failure to shoulder responsibility and other behavior reminiscent of a child, are also less inclined to feel sexual with someone who "acts like a child." When sexual frequency and enjoyment diminishes, both partners feel on edge, and other previously enjoyable aspects of the relationship may suffer. One of the biggest benefits to getting rid of the parent trap is more frequent and enjoyable sex. Many feel that this is a goal worth working toward!

You may ask, "What can I do when I feel that I have no other option but to nag, badger, or hassle my partner?" Keeping in mind that the goal is to disengage from toxic patterns and free yourself from the parent trap, the first step is to begin to recognize when you are coming across as parental. Be brutally honest as you reflect on the following questions:

- Do you use parental words or phrases to try to motivate your partner? If you heard someone else speaking in the same manner, what would you think?

- How are your words delivered? Is your tone of voice angry or harsh?

- Try to imagine how your body language and facial expression might look. What do your nonverbal gestures communicate to your partner?

After one of my clients became aware that she was taking on the role of a parent with her partner with ADHD and treating him like a disobedient child, she shared that she had spent their entire family vacation biting the inside of her lip to keep from saying the parental things she had become accustomed to saying to him. While I wouldn't recommend biting your lip as a solution, it is important to heighten your own awareness of the parent-child dynamic by taking a good look at what is going on with you and your partner.

The antidote to communicating as a parent is to communicate as an adult, which means that your words express what you need or feel. The best way to communicate as an adult is to begin practicing assertive communication. Assertive communication is a way of expressing your own needs and wants in a manner that is direct and honest, not hostile or mean. The partner who says, "I can't *believe* you are late again! What is *wrong* with you? How could you *do* this? You are *never* on time! You embarrass me *every time* we have to go somewhere," with an intense facial expression, a derisive tone of voice, and hands on hips is operating in angry, punitive parent mode.

Assertive Communication

The assertive way to express frustration is to use "I" statements. Although we discussed "I" statements in the previous chapter, it's worth a refresher course. Replacing the angry outburst with an "I" statement sounds something like this: "When I realize that you will be late again, I feel disrespected by you and would appreciate it if you would pay more attention to this, because it really, really bothers me." You may be laughing at me right now, saying, "Right, that'll work." I can't promise that it will work magically to get your partner to do what you are asking. What it will do is allow you to stop your participation in the toxic parent-child dynamic of the parent trap. As a result, you will feel better about yourself. There will be less wear and tear on your emotions, and you will be able to keep your focus on the problem, because it won't get diverted and become all about your angry response.

REHEARSING YOUR "I" STATEMENTS

You can get better at assertive communication by reflecting on past situations and thinking about how you could have handled your response differently. There will be moments in the future with your ADHD partner when you will become frustrated with one thing or another, so I suggest that you practice a dialogue with yourself. Reenact a recent situation in your head, but this time, speak your assertive response out loud; actually say the words. The purpose is to become more comfortable with how the words actually sound as they come out of your mouth. As you begin to formulate your "I" statements by saying them out loud, a good time to rehearse might be when you are alone and driving your car. Listen to how your voice sounds, and bring down the emotionality in the tone. Speak softer. Think about different phrases and approaches. Take a typical situation and construct "I" statements around it. Prepare for what you will do the next time a trying situation comes up.

AVOIDING ABSOLUTES

Try to stay away from absolutes. Using "never," as in "You never remember what I tell you," and "always," as in "You always forget what I've said," will usually produce a defensive response from your partner with ADHD, because you come across as judgmental. Even if it is true that your partner always forgets and never remembers, try to use different phrasing that incorporates "I" statements. Some good alternatives to absolutes are:

- *"More often than not,* I feel that you don't listen to me."

- *"It seems that a lot of the time,* what I say is forgotten."

- *"Frequently,* I feel unheard."

PLAYING THE BROKEN RECORD

You can incorporate "I" statements into another assertive communication skill, *playing the broken record,* which means repeating your point over and over again. Sticking to your point, regardless of your partner's response, will make you less likely to go off target and therefore less likely to fall into the parent trap. Using calm, repetitive statements enables you to control the tone of the interaction, which helps keep the dialogue focused on the problem that needs to be resolved.

Whenever my husband with ADHD drives, he has a tendency to change lanes without using his turn signal. I found that I got very upset whenever I was in the car with him, because I felt that this habit wasn't safe. I tended to use all of the unhealthy parent-trap devices to try to get him to use his turn signal: I would nag, berate, get angry, or use strong nonverbal gestures. My blood pressure would rise, I was miserable, and we would usually end up in an argument. After arriving at our destination, it would take me a while to shift my mood and be able to enjoy the outing.

Then one day I had a long talk with myself and decided to do things differently in the future. I came up with a plan. The next time we were in the car together and he didn't use the turn signal when changing lanes, I very calmly and matter-of-factly said, "You know, I get nervous when you don't use the turn signal when you change lanes, so when I am in the car with you, I would appreciate your using it." That was it—no lecture, no exasperated exclamations, no pleading tone in my voice. If I remember correctly, when I asked the first time, he responded tersely, but I held my ground and didn't engage or respond at all. A few minutes later I noticed that he had failed to use the turn signal again (which I knew would happen), so I was ready. I calmly played the broken record by saying, "I would like it if you would use your turn signal when I'm in the car with you." His response was edgy; still accustomed to my parental approach, he responded in his usual manner. Anyway, I held my ground. We had several more rounds of my asking calmly, assertively, and in an adult manner for him to please use the turn signal when I was in the car with him. He finally said, "Oh, all right!" with an attitude. But guess what? He used the turn signal from then on without my having to say another thing about it! There was no argument; we avoided falling fully into the parent trap, and I arrived at our destination calm and composed.

Your partner's ADHD is not going to go away. It will remain a constant. There will always be behaviors and attitudes that have the potential to create relational roadblocks. But I encourage you to keep up your effort to create healthier ways to interact with your partner, handle your frustrations, and communicate your feelings. It is your responsibility to decide how you want to communicate and to conduct yourself so that you stop participating in the parent trap. Diminishing your parental role is a crucial, necessary step for the future of your relationship.

CHAPTER 10

Taking Care of Yourself

Recently, while standing in the grocery checkout line, I surveyed the magazines on display and was surprised at how many articles promoted the issue of *self-care*. Headlines such as "10 Ways to Incorporate Good Self-Care into Your Busy Life" and "Slow Down, Chill Out: Take Care of You!" filled the magazine covers. Since I am an advocate of good self-care, I was curious to see if the subject was as popular as the magazines made it out to be, so at home, I did an online search for the word "self-care," which resulted in thousands of references to the subject.

What exactly does self-care mean, why is it so important, and how do you do it? For most people, it means taking time out of a busy day or week to devote time and effort to an endeavor that offers physical, mental, or emotional restoration. Ideally, good self-care provides our bodies, minds, and emotions with renewed energy to help us perform ordinary daily tasks at optimal levels and to enable us to handle all of life's stressors that come our way. And while there are lots of options for implementing self-care habits in our lives, there is no one-size-fits-all solution; it's based on individual preferences and personal inclinations: one person may like to rock climb, while another prefers to meditate in a quiet room.

Why You Need to Add Good Self-Care to Your Life

Good self-care provides a balance in life that helps to offset the stressors and trials of everyday living. While it is important for everyone to apply good self-care principles, it is vitally important that you, as the non-ADHD partner, be especially attentive to this. The challenges involved in living with your ADHD partner's distractibility, impulsivity, procrastination, poor follow-through, and restlessness, to name a few, can rob you of time and other resources that you could use for self-care and self-fulfillment. Many of the non-ADHD partners whom I work with in my therapy practice have lost touch with good self-care habits, because their lives get wrapped up in taking care of the partner who has ADHD. One of my priorities in our counseling sessions is to help the non-ADHD partner to become more mindful of ways to incorporate healthy activities and new habits that will benefit the body, mind, and emotions.

A healthy approach to your physical, mental, and emotional well-being will result in more peace and contentment in your personal life and, consequently, a more satisfying and fulfilling relational life. The next time you are on an airplane, pay attention to the flight attendant's instructions for using the oxygen mask should it become necessary: you are told to put on your own oxygen mask before trying to help others. The reason for these instructions is simple: if you suffer from a lack of oxygen, your body will fail and then you won't be able to help anyone around you. In much the same way, personal self-care is similar to the airplane oxygen mask: if you fail to find time to practice a reasonable amount of good self-care that renews and refreshes you, you will have less physical, mental, and emotional energy to be of any help or assistance to others in your life, especially your partner who has ADHD.

• Sylvia and Her Partner with ADHD

One non-ADHD client, named Sylvia, recently complained to me that she felt as though all of her extra time and energy were used to ensure that her ADHD partner did the things he needed to do. She said that she began every day by thinking about each of her responsibilities and each of his responsibilities for that day. As the day progressed, she started wondering whether her partner had accomplished, or would accomplish, his responsibilities. (His responsibilities were not significant but involved simple things, such as remembering to be on time when picking up their son from school or starting dinner preparations when he arrived home.)

Over time, Sylvia had discovered that the best plan was to check in with him during the day so that she could put her mind to rest. That seems easy enough, but for Sylvia it wasn't quite that simple. Because she knew that her partner with ADHD struggled with distractibility, she felt that she had to spend extra time and energy each day deciding exactly when to check in with him so that she could gently remind him of his daily responsibilities. She learned that if she checked in too early in the day, there was a strong possibility that he would forget the task because of his tendency to go offtrack with all of the inevitable distractions that came his way. She also knew that if she checked in too late, she ran the risk that he had already forgotten and was completely involved in something else that would result in her having to stop whatever she was doing to pick up their son or scramble to buy food for dinner. One of Sylvia's main complaints was that much of her extra energy during the course of a day was spent determining the optimal time to contact her partner and making time in her schedule to do it.

Sylvia is a good example of a non-ADHD partner focusing her own physical and mental energy toward managing her partner who has ADHD. When I asked her what she might do with those extra minutes in her day that she used to plan and carry out follow-up with her partner, she responded that, although she had not thought about it in a long time, maybe she would put her feet up in the afternoon and have a cup of tea or take time to read an interesting article, both excellent self-care activities that had disappeared from her life. After Sylvia realized that she had forsaken her self-care for a long time to deal with this issue, she had a heart-to-heart talk with her partner about her feelings. Fortunately, he responded positively, and together they had a brainstorming session to find a new solution to the dilemma.

Your Body and Emotions

Losing good self-care habits while in relationship with your partner who has ADHD can bring dire consequences: your body and mind can wear out, resulting in physical problems, emotional exhaustion, or both. The somatic, or bodily, problems that can arise are headaches, muscle aches, gastrointestinal problems, and worse. A colleague once confided in me that, although she couldn't prove it, she believed that her immune system disorder was partly due to the stress and strain of living for over twenty-five years with her partner who had ADHD.

Dysthymia

In addition to physical complaints, it's not unusual for the non-ADHD partner to have a depressed mood, particularly if good self-care activities aren't factored into daily living. The type of depression that I have observed most frequently in the non-ADHD partner isn't the type depicted on television commercials that tout antidepressant medications—you know, the ads that show a forlorn, lethargic person dragging through the day. That type of depression is called *major depressive disorder* (MDD). Less severe than MDD and therefore harder to recognize is another type of depression, called *dysthymia*. Dysthymia is characterized by a chronic depressed state that can last for many years, and while it has the same characteristics as MDD, it doesn't result in the same degree of impairment in daily life. The person with dysthymia is able to work and carry out daily activities, but often feels as though he is just going through the motions. Dysthymia is similar to a pesky fly or gnat that keeps buzzing and circling overhead: it never causes enough of a disturbance to get out the flyswatter but is problematic and irritating all the same, mainly because it never seems to go away.

Take a moment to read through the following list of symptoms that describe dysthymia, based on the *DSM-IV-TR* (APA 2000):

- Prolonged depressed mood

- Two or more of the following symptoms:

- sense of hopelessness about the future

- poor self-perception

- trouble concentrating or making decisions

- diminished physical energy or tendency to feel fatigued

- sleeping too much or too little

- either a lack of appetite or eating too much

If you feel that you meet the criteria for dysthymia or are headed in that direction, talk to your doctor or health care professional. Left untreated, dysthymia can spiral into a major depressive disorder, which can have significant personal and relational consequences.

Anxiety

Anxiety is another condition that non-ADHD partners commonly experience, especially when there is no effort to incorporate good self-care practices. Anxiety, a hyperawareness of the environment, occurs when your mind is in a constant state of arousal. This constant state of arousal creates a sense of danger and the feeling that something might happen that will require a quick response. So the mind tells the body to be on alert, to be ready and prepared all the time. As with depression, there are different types of anxiety: *generalized anxiety disorder* is commonly explained as "excessive worrying," worrying about everything or focusing on what could go wrong. The non-ADHD partner is very susceptible to generalized anxiety and is often accused of being a worry-wart, when the truth is that she has learned that she needs to be hypervigilant and aware because she may be called on to help her partner out of a predicament at any given time.

PANIC DISORDER

A more acute state of anxiety results in *panic disorder*, which tends to materialize out of the blue and has strong physical symptoms that can be frightening. Jeremy is a good example.

• Jeremy and His Partner with ADHD

Jeremy's situation with his wife who had ADHD could have contributed to his severe state of anxiety, resulting in a panic attack. Jeremy's wife had a habit of impulsively spending too much money and, due to her distractibility, would often forget to transfer money to cover her expenditures. Added to this dilemma was the fact that Jeremy's job required him to travel a lot so that he wasn't around to monitor what was happening with their bank account on a regular basis.

Before every trip, Jeremy set aside time to talk to his wife about being more careful and accountable with their money, especially while he was out of town. Although she was amenable, she would often forget his admonitions about her spending habits and buy something she "had to have," get distracted by something else, and then forget to make sure the bank account was covered or to let Jeremy know about her purchases. So while Jeremy tried hard to cross all of his "t's" and dot all of his "i's," he would regularly discover that their shared account had gone into overdraft, causing extra charges, or he would get a call from his credit card company because his wife had taken their credit to the limit again, affecting their credit profile. This common scenario left him scrambling to transfer money to avoid penalties and fees while on a business trip, when his time and availability were limited. Once he had handled the crisis, he began to dread his return home, because he knew he would have to have another serious talk with his wife about her spending and how this ongoing problem inconvenienced him. Jeremy didn't like playing the role of the heavy; he loved his wife and desired a mutually satisfying and fulfilling relationship with her.

One day, out of the blue, Jeremy felt pounding in his chest and tightness in his throat, and found it hard to take a breath. Frightened, he found the nearest emergency facility, because he was sure that he was having a heart attack. Over the following weeks, his doctor put him through all kinds of tests but couldn't find anything wrong. Jeremy finally realized that he was in a constant state of anxiety, fearful that his wife was going to lead them to financial ruin. He also realized that he had experienced the common symptoms of anxiety for the past few years: he was constantly tense, worried, and on edge, and found that these feelings interfered with his ability to fully enjoy his life. He also had an increasing sense that something bad or dangerous was imminent, especially when he felt out of control financially, which was often. Despite his job security and comfortable salary, the anxiety attached to this dilemma caused his thoughts to become irrational, and he often imagined himself penniless and homeless in the near future.

The stress of his financial predicament, caused by his wife's ADHD symptoms of impulsivity and distractibility, had gotten the better of him, and he was always anxious or worried—prior to his trip, while he was away, and right after he returned. Jeremy's anxiety connected to his wife's ADHD interfered with the quality of his life and the quality of his relationship with his wife. He realized that most of his mental and emotional energy was spent on his concerns regarding this issue, and he also discovered that he had completely given up on the activities and interests that used to bring him some relief from his anxious thoughts. He had dropped out of his weekly basketball game with his buddies at the Y, and he didn't even know where his camera was anymore. A big part of treating his anxiety was to help him make some healthy, positive changes in his life, including better self-care. He started playing basketball again and regularly took time on Saturday mornings to go hiking and photograph wildlife.

Depression and anxiety rob people of the ability to live life fully, yet are common consequences of the chronic frustration and disappointment that many non-ADHD partners experience as a result of being in a relationship with someone who has ADHD. To avoid falling into a deep, significant state of emotional distress, it is important to be aware of the warning signs and to take steps to prevent the situation from becoming worse.

Relational Burnout

We can't have a discussion about a relationship involving ADHD without examining the issue of *relational burnout* for the non-ADHD partner. Because of the tendency to overhelp, to become overinvolved, and to take over too many responsibilities in the relationship, the non-ADHD partner may expend too much physical and emotional energy, and, as a result, neglect her own physical, mental, and emotional needs and desires. The body and mind can't be on full alert forever without some relief; something has to give: the person gets tired or sick, and feels like giving up, a condition called burnout. While the normal demands of any relationship take a lot of effort, a relationship involving ADHD presents a greater possibility for the non-ADHD partner to become tapped out physically, mentally, and emotionally, thus interfering with the ability to be fully present and available for the relationship. Due to feeling stressed and overwhelmed, the non-ADHD partner finds that there are fewer positive moments and pleasurable activities in the relationship, and over time the connection between the couple weakens.

Relational burnout is a serious situation, and recovery can be difficult if too much damage has been done. The dynamics of relational burnout are very similar to those of caregiver burnout. A caregiver is usually a family member who regularly looks after another family member who has fallen ill or is incapacitated for some reason. The caregiver not only tends to the physical condition of the family member but also manages everything else: the home, the property, the finances, and all of the day-to-day problems that arise. While caring for a needy family member is an honorable endeavor, it also can be exhausting and stressful because of all of the responsibilities involved. And a very common consequence of caregiving is to become physically and emotionally depleted, causing the caregiver to be less effective at helping. The symptoms of relational burnout are similar to those associated with caregiver burnout.

- Feeling fatigued or less energetic than usual

- Being impatient and irritable with others

- Feeling sad or hopeless

- Feeling trapped by circumstances

- Isolating yourself from others

- Neglecting your own needs

- Feeling a loss of joy

- Getting physically sick more often

- Feeling overwhelmed by everyday demands

- Feeling unmotivated

Comparing the dynamics involved in caregiver burnout with the dynamics of ADHD relational burnout is worth further examination. The non-ADHD partner often attends to or takes care of the partner who has ADHD by managing the home, the family, and the environment because, in many situations, the symptoms of ADHD diminish the ADHD partner's ability to accomplish these tasks. This might include making sure that food is available and meals are prepared; providing a safe and clean home, both inside and out; managing the finances; running all of the errands; and taking care of children's needs. A caregiver who spends too much energy handling too many responsibilities without taking a break can get burned out. Similarly, when the non-ADHD partner becomes overwhelmed from handling too many jobs or duties without any support or assistance—especially from an able-bodied partner who has ADHD—then relationship burnout can result. This condition leaves significantly diminished energy for enjoyable activities; causes irritation toward the partner with ADHD; and perhaps leads to a sense of hopelessness, the feeling that life will never change for the better, resulting in less desire to put forth any effort at all. A downward spiral can occur, carrying the non-ADHD partner further and further into a feeling of despair about the relationship.

Caretaker burnout develops from the tendency to put the needs of those who are being cared for ahead of any needs the caregiver has. As with the well-meaning caretaker, it is common for the non-ADHD partner to put the needs of the partner with ADHD ahead of any personal needs. Keith, a man married to a woman with ADHD, described his life as "putting out one ADHD wildfire after another" and further complained that he was left with too little time to take care of his own needs. He said his wife's script ran something like this: "I forgot _____, and it needs to be taken care of immediately or else _____ will happen, and I don't have the time; can you take care of it?" Keith felt that if he didn't drop everything he was doing to take care of the chore or responsibility, there would be disastrous consequences; so he did drop everything that he was doing, often at the expense of his own responsibilities and desires. The end result was that her needs trumped his needs, and he took care of everything. His warning signs of burnout—feeling irritable, resentful, hopeless, and overwhelmed, and neglecting his own needs—were a wakeup call to face having to make some changes in his life.

For a caregiver, burnout doesn't happen overnight. The demands mount up day after day until the caregiver feels as if she were drowning with no life preserver in sight. Similarly, ADHD relational burnout occurs over time because one partner falls into patterns of overdoing and the other into a pattern of overdepending. The non-ADHD partner tends to take on more and more responsibility and to ignore the symptoms of burnout. Gradual changes can result in significant outcomes. One day the non-ADHD partner realizes that she is doing way more than she should, that she is burned out and fed up, and she says, "How the heck did I get myself into this?" Feeling exhausted, trapped, and hopeless, the non-ADHD partner may find herself in a potentially dangerous situation where she wants to just give up and walk away from the relationship.

• Martha

Martha was a textbook example of someone experiencing relational burnout. She and her husband with ADHD had married young. She worked and took care of their home affairs while he attended graduate school—for seven years! She didn't mind, she said, because she felt that her efforts and sacrifices were worth it for their future. After his graduation, she helped him compose his résumé and was very excited for him to find a job so that she could let go of some of her responsibilities. His job hunt took longer than she had anticipated, partly because he didn't seem very motivated, preferring to pursue all of his varied interests instead. He eventually did find employment, and Martha was relieved. But then their twins came along, which was when her life really began to fall apart. Her husband was not very helpful with the babies, and Martha soon found that she was taking care of everyone except herself. She continued to work part-time; take care of their finances; and do all of the shopping, cooking, cleaning, and child care. She increasingly complained to her husband but found that her complaints seemed to fall on deaf ears. In any case they didn't get her the desired response, which was for him to help her out. Little by little she took on the majority of responsibilities for their home and family life, because she felt that it was more of a hassle for her to repeatedly ask, remind, and wait for him to accomplish what she had requested. She couldn't remember the last time she had had the time to do even the smallest amount of self-care. After fifteen years of this type of marriage, she was at the end of her rope, and the only alternative she could imagine was to leave her husband. She did everything anyway, so what difference would it make?

How many of the symptoms of burnout apply to you? Do you feel fatigued or less energetic than usual? Are you impatient and irritable with others? Do you find yourself resentful and angry toward your partner who has ADHD? Do you feel hopeless that any changes will occur in the future? Have you lost connections with friends and others? Are you sick more often than previously? Are you experiencing more emotional breakdowns? Do you feel like saying, "What's the use?" If you answered yes to most of these questions, then you meet the criteria for relational burnout.

It's important to consider the severity of relational burnout. Rating levels of discomfort is a good indicator of the reality of our circumstances, and doing so can inform us that we may need to take some action. To illustrate this, I'm reminded of a recent visit to a friend who was in the hospital recovering from surgery. Every few hours a nurse would come in and ask my friend to rate her level of pain or discomfort on a scale from 0 to 10, with 0 meaning no pain at all and 10 meaning the most pain imaginable. If my friend reported a high number, then that would indicate that more medication was in order.

Using this model, take a moment to rate your symptoms on the Relational Burnout Scale. Doing so will help you get a clearer understanding of exactly what your discomfort level is and whether or not you need to take action. A quick overview of the warning signs of burnout will help you to assign the appropriate number: fatigue or diminished energy; impatience and irritability; resentment and anger toward your partner who has ADHD; hopelessness; isolation from friends and others; somatic problems, such as sickness and aches and pains; emotional volatility; and lack of motivation.

EXERCISE 10.1 THE RELATIONAL BURNOUT SCALE: Where Are You?

A rating of 0 or 1 on the Relational Burnout Scale means that everything in your relationship is great and you have no complaints (why are you reading this book, then?). A rating of 9 or 10 means that things are really bad, that you have answered yes to almost all of the symptoms of relational burnout, and that you might be considering walking away from your relationship. Any rating above 5 could indicate that you are falling into unhealthy patterns.

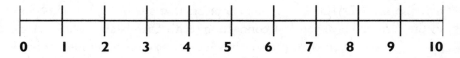

0   1   2   3   4   5   6   7   8   9   10

Regardless of how severe your rating is on the Relational Burnout Scale, it's never too late to begin undoing unhealthy patterns that are in place or are developing. One of the simplest and easiest methods for bringing that number on the Relational Burnout Scale down is to begin paying serious attention to better self-care. By doing this, you can actually offset some of the difficulties caused by relational burnout, even reversing the effects of depression and anxiety. Remember Martha and how desperate she felt? Once she realized how badly she had neglected herself, she started to incorporate better methods of self-care into her life and was determined to put on her own "oxygen mask" first. The end result was that she began to feel better about herself and then felt more connected to her partner and her family.

Good Self-Care

Basic self care begins with the body: food is fuel for your body, so watch what you eat and drink. It's essential to maintain a balanced diet filled with healthy foods and to drink lots of water. It's just as important to limit sugar, caffeine, and alcohol intake. How would you rate your habits in this area? Are there any changes that you need to make? Physical activity is another basic tenet of good self-care. When was the last time you exercised? Why did you stop? What would it take for you to begin again?

Good self-care is just as important for the mind: at the simplest level, this means getting enough sleep. Sleep is designed to reboot our brains so that we can feel refreshed and renewed the next day. Without it, you can't function at the best of your ability. How well do you sleep? Do you rely on drugs or alcohol to help you sleep? Do you have good sleep hygiene?

Emotional self-care can't be ignored, yet many non-ADHD part-ners have walled off their emotions and lost touch with recognizing and expressing their emotional states. Rather than feel and experience all emotions, the non-ADHD partner doesn't allow any and may come across as flat and detached, seemingly not caring about anything at all. Have you shut off your emotions? Are you afraid that all you can feel is anger? When was the last time you remember feeling joy or contentment?

Good self-care is a subjective experience. Not all people will be ener-gized and renewed in the same way. My idea of good self-care is to enjoy a really good book, while my husband prefers a vigorous bike ride in the mountains. It really doesn't matter what you do, as long as you commit to incorporating some beneficial activities into your life. The following self-care activities list is designed to give you some suggestions that will help you to avoid relational burnout or to find your way back from it. Use some of the ideas on the list or make up some of your own.

SELF-CARE ACTIVITY LIST

- Do something creative: learn how to sketch, draw, paint, knit, or crochet, for example.

- Take time to relax and pamper yourself; put your feet up for a few minutes every day.

- Have a cup of tea or coffee with a friend or by yourself.

- Get a massage.

- Take a bubble bath.

- Get a manicure and pedicure.

- Take an acting class (an excellent way of getting in touch with your feelings).

- Check out a good book from the library and set aside some time to read.

- Put on headphones and listen to music.

- Dance.

- Exercise your body; recommit to some physical activity that you enjoyed in the past.

- Look for a new activity, such as a spinning class or a kick-boxing class (good for getting out aggression).

- Try Pilates or yoga (good for calming and centering the emotions).

- Take up golf.

- Pick up a magazine or newspaper.

- If you don't have any money for classes, then put on your tennis shoes and start walking or running with a friend or alone; just get moving.

- Find some fellowship: reach out to friends; reconnect with old ones or meet some new ones.

- Attend classes to learn something new: a language, cooking, or some other skill.

- Find enjoyable activities with other like-minded people.

- Go to a museum.

- Attend religious services.

- Find (or start) a support group for non-ADHD partners.

- Sit outside in the sunshine.

- Take a nap.

- Pray or meditate.

- Start a journal and write about your feelings.

- Look up at the stars in the sky at night.

- Watch a movie that you've wanted to see or revisit an old favorite.

- Light a fragrant candle.

- Find something to laugh at.

As you can see, good self-care doesn't have to be complicated or cost a lot of money; all it requires is your effort and time.

Appropriate Selfishness

When I encounter a non-ADHD client who has an ADHD partner and appears to be depressed or anxious, or possibly suffering from relationship burnout, I usually start by asking the person what he is doing to take care of himself. After the client stops laughing, we begin an earnest discussion of the benefits of good self-care. I explain that the demands in a relationship involving ADHD can be taxing, and I emphasize that it is essential to incorporate healthy self-care activities to be better equipped to ward off depression, anxiety, or relational deterioration. I verbally challenge my client to become *appropriately selfish*. I explain that *appropriate* selfishness is a very positive and healthy concept. It means that you give yourself permission to state what your needs are and that you take positive steps to get them met; you take time to pay attention to what your mind and body are telling you; you decide what feels good (and what doesn't); and you invest time, energy, and resources toward bringing healthy changes to your life—all without guilt.

The challenge to integrate appropriate selfishness into life can be a difficult concept, because "selfish" is perceived as a dirty word that means too much concentration and focus on oneself. But changing the way we view "selfish" is critical for finding new ways to navigate life. While doing so may require a real shift in thinking, the end result is that you will feel better about yourself and be more available for your relationship. By incorporating appropriate selfishness, you will have more energy to focus on your partner's needs and will be able to meet those needs in a more meaningful and authentic way. You won't be operating out of a deficit anymore, because appropriate selfishness incorporates all the elements of good self-care: diet, adequate sleep, exercise, and vitalizing activities. I challenge you to become appropriately selfish.

Are you convinced yet of the far-reaching benefits of developing good self-care habits? Did you ever think that watching a couple of episodes of *I Love Lucy*, having a cup of tea, or taking a walk around the block could be so meaningful? Are you fully aware of the dire consequences that can occur as a result of omitting good self-care from your life? A life of depression and anxiety robs you of joy and contentment. Relational burnout creates loneliness and isolation. Your day-to-day life with your partner who has ADHD may be distressing, frustrating, and trying, but I urge you to begin taking better care of yourself. It's your job; no one else will do it for you.

CHAPTER 11

Moving through Obstacles Together

If you listen carefully to love songs or read love poems, you will notice a common theme. As the singers and poets sing and speak eloquently about love, they all seem thrilled with the prospect of joining together with a partner so that they will never feel lonely again. Most of us share the same hopes and dreams of togetherness when we commit to a relationship. But living with a partner who has ADHD can, at times, be a very lonely experience. Because of distractibility, restlessness, and inattention, ADHD has a way of taking the "us" out of a relationship and creating a "you versus me" dynamic. The you versus me feeling can bring unique challenges to the relationship that are harmful and damaging, resulting in hurt feelings, resentment, and bitterness. In fact, research has shown that adults with ADHD are twice as likely to be divorced (Toner, O'Donoghue, and Houghton 2006).

The active symptoms of distractibility, restlessness, and impulsivity can spirit our partners with ADHD away, isolating them from those whom they love and care for the most. When this happens, we feel lonely—and also confused, angry, disappointed, and unhappy. We may wonder how we got ourselves into this. What's the saving grace, then? What keeps us around? Why do we stay? I ask this question of all of my clients who have a partner with ADHD, and here is the essence of how they respond: "It's because I know his heart; despite how much his behavior can hurt me, I know he isn't a mean-spirited person. I know that he doesn't ignore me intentionally, that he doesn't mean to be difficult when he gets up from the dinner table before I finish eating, and that carelessly spoken words or phrases weren't intended to wound me. In spite of how ADHD affects his behavior, I do believe he loves me, and in spite of how ADHD affects his behavior, I love him, too."

The antidote to the you versus me dilemma, and to the staggering divorce rate, is to take advantage of any opportunity that will help to strengthen your relationship. The previous chapters asked you to consider making some changes in your own attitudes and behaviors, including creating and maintaining healthy boundaries, using different approaches with your partner, learning how to manage anger, establishing good self-care habits, and recognizing potential relational pitfalls—all for the purpose of making the relationship healthier and stronger. It doesn't matter if you have been with your partner for three years or thirty; any effort you put forth toward these personal changes can help to minimize the harm that ADHD can create or has already created in your relationship.

If you have made it this far in the book and taken the time and effort to understand yourself better and to modify your reactions and responses to your partner for the purpose of strengthening your relationship, maybe your relationship with your partner with ADHD has become less stressful. It might be the time to enlist the aid of your partner for the purpose of strengthening your relationship *together*. Ideally, working together will create a stronger relational foundation and also provide protection for your relationship when, in the future, it may become necessary to confront new challenges. Creating a solid relational foundation doesn't happen overnight; it will require that you and your partner with ADHD, working as a team, engage in proactive, strategic preparation and planning. This chapter primarily focuses on exercises that are designed to help you build up and fortify your relationships.

Building a Strong Relational Foundation

The first step in building a strong relational foundation is to conduct a *SWOT analysis*: a planning method that businesses use to help their companies identify key areas of *strengths, weaknesses, opportunities,* and *threats*.

In many ways, a couple's relationship is similar to a business partnership. In a business partnership, there is usually a division of duties based on skills. Each partner has certain capabilities that contribute to the success of the business: one partner may be good at finances and organization, while the other is more of a visionary. While these divisions may not be intentionally created as in a business situation, this dynamic is often present in a relational partnership.

- In business, strategy meetings need to be held to examine the bottom line, make sound decisions, and plan for the future. Ongoing and open communication is also an important component in a relational partnership.

- In a business there should be a shared desire to make the partnership profitable so that everyone benefits from his or her labors. While no one gets a paycheck in a relational partnership, there are payoffs: goodwill, contentment, and satisfaction, to name a few.

So it's not too much of a stretch to adapt a business model to assess the health and well-being of a relationship.

EXERCISE 11.1 SWOT ANALYSIS

Your SWOT analysis will help you to identify your strengths and weaknesses as a couple and what opportunities might be available to you, and will help you to notice any possible threats to your relationship.

Step 1: Identify strengths. You will discover your relational strengths by realistically rating your level of satisfaction in certain areas. Read the following questions and rate them on a scale from 1 to 10, where 1 means extremely low, 5 means average, and 10 means extremely high. Any number from 7 up is considered a strength. Then compare your ratings with those of your partner. Note: This exercise is designed to bring clarity to your relationship, so if you find that you and your partner have vastly different responses, you will need to engage in deeper discussions. I caution you against becoming defensive, because it will defeat the purpose of the exercise.

_____ As an individual, how would you rate your satisfaction level in how you and your partner communicate?

_____ As an individual, how would you rate your satisfaction level in how you and your partner resolve conflicts?

_____ As an individual, how would you rate your satisfaction level in how you and your partner make decisions?

_____ As an individual, how would you rate your satisfaction level in how you and your partner manage money?

_____ As an individual, how would you rate your satisfaction level in your sexual intimacy with your partner?

_____ As an individual, how would you rate your satisfaction level in how you spend your free time together?

_____ As an individual, how would you rate your satisfaction level in how you and your partner divide duties?

_____ As an individual, how would you rate your satisfaction level in how you and your partner parent (only if applicable)?

After completing this part of the exercise, discuss the following questions with your partner:

- *What strengths are easily recognizable?*

- *Are there any surprises?*

- *Do we have any strengths that are not mentioned?*

- *Is there anything that either of us can do as individuals to maximize our strengths?*

- *Is there anything that we can do as a couple to maximize our strengths?*

Step 2: Identify weaknesses. Once you have identified your strengths in the relationship, you will be able to easily identify your weaknesses by examining the areas that you rated the lowest (anything below 5). Don't be discouraged if you have several areas of weakness; it's not unusual. It's important to examine the weaknesses by discussing the following questions:

- *Are there any weaknesses that are surprising to either of us?*

- *Are there any that could be detrimental to our relationship?*

- *Is there anything that either of us can do as individuals to minimize our weaknesses?*

- *Is there anything that we can do as a couple to minimize our weaknesses?*

After your discussion of possible weaknesses, make a list of the areas that you rated as lower than 5. From this list you will create at least one "we" statement for each item. A "we" statement is a declaration of intent for the future. For instance, if you scored low on communication, your "we" statement might be We *could communicate better if we set aside some time every week to compare our calendars and talk about what is going on.* Or it you scored low in sexual intimacy, a beneficial "we" statement could be We *would have more opportunity for sex if we went to bed at the same time every night.* "We" statements are constructive attempts to find solutions to your areas of weakness.

Step 3: Identify opportunities. This segment of the analysis is designed to help you discover what is already happening within your relationship or what could possibly occur in the future to enhance your relationship. I guided Jay and Charlene (the ADHD partner) through this process. Married for about four years, they had yet to start a family. I asked them what opportunities were available to them that could increase their relational well-being; here are some of their thoughts:

- *We are both smart and ambitious.*

- *Charlene is creative and imaginative.*

- *Jay is a hard worker.*

- *We both have marketable skills that will help us to stay employed.*

- *We share the same values.*

- *We have supportive families who love and care about us.*

- *We have a stable living environment.*

- *We want the same things out of life.*

- *We enjoy the same hobbies.*

- *We both have a sense of humor that allows us to laugh at ourselves and find humor in most things.*

As they listed all of their opportunities, they realized that they had taken a lot for granted in their relationship, which helped them to refocus on many of the positive aspects of their life together. This part of the analysis is the most pleasurable, because couples often begin to see the possibility of a brighter future.

Create a list of at least ten opportunities that might be available to you that would provide more satisfaction and fulfillment in your relationship. After listing your opportunities, discuss the following questions:

- *How can we, as a couple, maximize the opportunities that we have identified?*

- *How can we, as individuals, maximize the opportunities that we have identified?*

Step 4: Identify threats. Threats are any external forces or people that can cause stress to the relationship. Threats aren't necessarily intended to harm us, but are realistic circumstances that need to be recognized. Phyllis and James, a couple in their midfifties, completed this part of the exercise by including the following threats:

- *Health concerns as we grow older*

- *Fewer job opportunities*

- *The possibility that our oldest child will have to move back in with us*

- *Phyllis's unstable boss*

- *A depressed economy*

- *The possible need to become caretakers of elderly parents*

Some of their responses seem to be more individualized—for instance, Phyllis's unstable boss. When I asked how her boss created a threat to their relationship, Phyllis replied that her situation at work created so much stress that she often came home quite upset, which affected how the rest of their evening together was spent. While Phyllis and James didn't necessarily enjoy this part of the assignment, it did produce some positive results: previously they had put off going to the doctor, but as a result of examining potential threats that included future health concerns, they were motivated to schedule physical exams (and were found to be in excellent health).

After you make a list of the potential threats to your relationship, discuss the following questions:

- *Are there any threats to our relationship that can be eliminated?*

- *Are there any threats to our relationship that we could manage better?*

- *Is there anything that either of us can do as individuals to minimize the threats we have identified?*

- *Is there anything that we can do as a couple to minimize the threats we have identified?*

Determining Your Direction as a Couple

The following exercise is designed to help you, as a couple, decide which direction you want your life to go by creating *couple goals*. The biggest benefit to having mutually decided-on, clearly defined goals is that it can help you to make decisions on a daily basis. Without clear couple goals, time passes and couples find that they haven't achieved the things in life that they desired. Creating goals can be especially helpful in relationships involving ADHD, because it can diminish procrastination, as in, "Honey, remember that we decided to get our old car up and running this weekend so that we could sell it and put the money into our vacation account." Another benefit of couple goals is that the goal, not the non-ADHD partner, becomes the "boss" that says no to impulsive behaviors, such as spending money. Many positive outcomes can be gained from setting couple goals, including relational structure, purpose, and harmony.

EXERCISE 11.2 SETTING COUPLE GOALS

Based on the previous information that you acquired by completing your SWOT analysis, agree on some couple goals that will help make your relationship successful. The goals can be about anything: finances, your relationship, intimacy, family, and so on. But keep the following in mind: the goals should be fair, reasonable, and consistent with your values. They must also be quantifiable; in other words, put a value on the goal. How many days, months, or years will it take to achieve a particular goal? Don't just say, "'Someday' we will buy a house"; factor in all of the details and put a do-by date on each one. If the goal has to do with money, then give it a definable amount: "We want to save X amount of dollars by this time next year."

Next, categorize your goals as *short-term goals* and *long-term goals*. For instance, Mark and Celia's goals included taking a vacation to Costa Rica the following Christmas (short-term) but also included moving to Hawaii when they retired (long-term). After you have determined your short-term and long-term goals, the next step is to create *action steps* that will help you to accomplish them. For Mark and Celia to reach their goal of taking a vacation to Costa Rica, their first action step was to open a savings account specifically for that purpose. The next action step attached to that goal was to take a certain amount of money out of their paychecks each week and put it in the savings account. Mark knew that Celia, who had ADHD, would likely spend the money on less important things if they didn't create these action steps. For their long-term goal of moving to Hawaii when they retired, one of their action steps was to set up an appointment with a financial adviser so that they could begin planning for that time in their life together. Goals are harder to achieve without specific action steps to help accomplish them.

One important thing to remember is that your goals are living documents; they are not carved in stone, so be flexible. Life has a way of throwing curveballs at us, so remember that you may not be able to achieve a particular goal in the time you expected. Don't give up on the process, though; continue to review and renew your goals from time to time.

A Mission Statement

Many couples and families follow another business model by developing and adopting *personal mission statements*. Companies and other entities create mission statements to help define who they are and what they do. It also helps keep them focused on their purpose, why they exist. I experienced the value of a mission statement several years ago, when I served on the board of a nonprofit corporation. Many new ideas and concepts were introduced and discussed, but if we found that they weren't in line with our mission statement, we knew that they would ultimately take the organization away from its original purpose. A mission statement helps to pinpoint overall intentions, purposes, and priorities.

EXERCISE 11.3 DEVELOP YOUR MISSION STATEMENT

For you and your partner, developing a mission statement means identifying your vision for your relationship and your values. Some questions to consider when you create your mission statement are: What is important for you as a couple? How do you want to live your life together? How do you want to be regarded? What are your standards?

Karina and Sam had already worked through their SWOT analysis and then created their short-term and long-term couple goals, along with the appropriate action steps, and were now intrigued by the idea of creating a mission statement for their relationship. Here is what they came up with:

> We, Karina and Sam, commit to spending our lives together in order to authentically demonstrate fidelity, acceptance, loving care, and respect for each other so that we can serve as a healthy model for our families and our community.

> They had both come from highly dysfunctional families and felt that their mission statement not only created purpose and meaning for them but also kept them mindful of how they wanted to live their lives differently from what they had experienced in their families.

Changing How You Interact

As a result of the two of you working together to clarify your wants and needs in your relationship, you may find that in order to achieve more contentment, productivity, and effectiveness, some things need to change. If you are earnest about making those changes, the next challenge is to *examine your systems*, or the way you interact with each other.

Once again we can apply a business concept to relationships. Just as businesses have certain *systems* in place that run day-to-day operations, we all have personal ways, or systems, of doing everything in our lives, such as time management, finances, and meals. We have systems in place to handle even the most common behaviors; did you realize that you have your own system for getting out of bed in the morning? If a business becomes aware that a certain system isn't working well—if it could be better, faster, and more profitable—then the business will examine ways to change that system. The same is true with us: if a certain system isn't working, then we usually try to use other options, right? For instance, if your system for getting out of bed in the morning isn't working very well and you tend to oversleep, then it's a good idea to modify the system, perhaps by getting a new alarm clock that has a very loud buzzer and putting it across the room so that you have to get out of bed to turn it off. Better systems produce better outcomes.

Just as we have all kinds of systems in place for navigating the day, we also have systems in place for the more abstract areas of our lives, such as how we relate to and with our partners. So even though you may not be aware of it, you and your partner with ADHD have certain systems in place for communicating and resolving conflict with each other. If your relationship is typical of most couples involving ADHD, you may find that due to ADHD symptoms, such as distractibility, restlessness, and impulsivity, your systems might not be very healthy or productive. If you and your partner find that you often end up bickering, then you will need to examine how your systems of communication and conflict resolution may need to be changed to give you better outcomes.

By not giving proper attention to changing unhealthy systems, you may both find that you feel unduly stressed and are becoming more and more angry and irritable with each other. As one non-ADHD partner shared with me, "My spouse's inability to live much beyond *now* means that I often feel angry and 'put upon.' Our having such poor ability to communicate and resolve the problems has definitely changed the way I feel about our relationship." Trying to manage your own emotions while dealing with an ADHD partner's challenges can be wearisome and, as we have discovered, over time can build into a feeling of despair and a loss of hope, as this woman felt. If you find yourself in the same situation or feel that you are moving in that direction, it is time to examine your current relational system and consider the changes that can be made.

One aspect of my work with couples is to help them understand how all of the systems that are in place in their relationships may not be getting them desired results, such as relational peace and harmony. So we start by searching for more productive methods to enhance communication and resolve problems. One couple whom I treated was ready and willing, at least to some extent, to find a way to change a problematic situation in their marriage.

• Marilyn and Clark

Marilyn and Clark had been married for about fifteen years when they sought my services. Clark had hyperactive-impulsive type ADHD, and many areas of their family life could be described as a roller coaster, consisting of considerable ups and downs.

Marilyn and Clark did a SWOT analysis and, as a result, began to prioritize the changes that they wanted to make in their relationship. They both agreed that Clark's poor time management was one of their biggest challenges. Over the years, Marilyn had developed the ability to separate herself from how Clark managed his own affairs, but whenever his lack of punctuality affected her life, she continued to feel irate and angry about it. Furthermore, although Clark indicated that he knew time management was a problem for him, he seemed to be able to roll with the punches and remain unbothered whenever the couple was late. Marilyn, however, would steam and stew about it for hours, and quite often the event or occasion was ruined for her.

They decided to target one specific system in their life together concerning Clark's poor time management, to see if they could make any change. After making the necessary change, they would see if it brought about positive results. Marilyn said that one of her most trying situations was being late to church every week because Clark was never ready to leave on time. Marilyn wanted to arrive early so that she could feel calm and centered before the service began. She said that because Clark was never ready on time despite his awareness of how important it was to her, she felt significantly disrespected by him.

They recounted how Sunday mornings usually went: First Marilyn would begin to remind Clark of the time. He tended to wave her off with a "Yeah, yeah, I'll be ready on time." A slow burn would grow as the time to leave got closer and she noticed that Clark wasn't ready. As the minutes ticked by, the slow burn boiled over, and Marilyn would explode in anger. Marilyn's anger got Clark's attention and served the purpose of providing him with enough adrenaline to be able to focus on the task at hand. He would then rush around in a frenzy and finally be ready to leave. In the car on the way to church, Marilyn would either continue to complain about the situation or sit in stony silence (which is another strong communication gesture). Clark would take offense at her angry complaints or her stony silence, and an argument would ensue all the way until they reached the parking lot. Clark said he was usually able to shake it off, but Marilyn would often be in tears as they walked up to the front door of the church. They both felt that this too-familiar scenario was counterproductive to their purpose in going to church.

The reality was that Marilyn and Clark's system for getting to church wasn't working at all; in fact, it was doing a lot of damage to their relationship. The solution was to come up with a different system for Sunday mornings that would allow both Marilyn and Clark to feel calm and peaceful, rather than angry and upset at each other. They examined all possible options and finally decided that, rather than wait for Clark on Sunday mornings, Marilyn would take her own car to church if Clark was running late. This new system would allow her to arrive before the service began, which was what she desired. While Clark needed to be convinced that this new approach would create a much better final outcome—he really didn't feel that being late was that big of a deal—he decided that he would go along with the new solution. They were both determined to make this change happen, so they put the new plan into action.

The next time I met with them, they reported that the new system was working well. Clark didn't like going to church alone, but did confess that Marilyn seemed "less bothered" when she went ahead on her own. "Less bothered" was the understatement of the year: Marilyn had told me that she had been considering leaving Clark over this. Marilyn was more than happy to ride to church with Clark if he was ready on time without a lot of input (that is, complaining) from her. But she held firm on their new plan that she would take her car and go on her own when he ran late. She found that she felt much better on an emotional level. "I don't have any anger toward Clark, and therefore I'm much more pleasant to be around," she observed. He agreed!

Another benefit to this newly created system was that Marilyn gave up the responsibility of making Clark leave the house at a particular time. This system appropriately returned to Clark the task of putting more effort into being ready on time so that he didn't have to depend on Marilyn's anger to motivate him. Successfully changing this system gave both of them the encouragement that they needed to address other systems that were creating problems in their relationship.

EXERCISE 11.4 EXAMINE YOUR SYSTEMS

The following is the formula Marilyn and Clark used to figure out how to change their system and come up with a new one:

1. Target the problem; find one area that continues to be habitually problematic in your relationship.

2. Make a list of *all* possible solutions. Don't make any comments or ridicule any of them; just get them all on the table.

3. Discuss each possibility, including its pros and cons.

4. Pick one new solution to try. Put it in place.

5. Afterward, have a debriefing. Did it go as expected? Did it fail? Are there any adjustments that need to be made? Do you need to choose another solution to try?

It was easy for Marilyn and Clark to find a problem to fix, since this one had created difficulty for them for many years. They had fun coming up with a list of other possible solutions: go to church in separate cars all the time, stop going to church at all, find a church with a later service, and have Clark set his alarm earlier on Sunday mornings (Marilyn had to keep from laughing out loud at that one). The solution that they chose, go to church in separate cars when Clark was not ready in time, seemed to be the one that worked for them. After a couple of weeks, they talked the matter over again and decided that this was still the best solution for them, because they discovered that as feelings of goodwill and respect replaced the anger and arguments, they both felt better.

Forgiveness

The following exercise is a complete departure from the previous ones, switching from a business model to an intensely private and emotional model of how to forgive. You may find yourself at a crossroads in your relationship with your partner who has ADHD, and you may be experiencing a wide range of strong negative emotions. During the course of your relationship, your partner's ADHD symptoms might have caused you to feel neglected, disrespected, misunderstood, unsupported, invalidated, and underappreciated. This book has tried to put ADHD in perspective for you and help you understand that ADHD is a neurobiological disorder, that it can affect every dimension of a person's life, and that it especially affects relationships. As the non-ADHD partner, you are the person who lives most intimately with your partner who has ADHD; you get to experience the intensity of his ADHD more than anyone else. While your rational mind knows that the ADHD-influenced behavior isn't usually intentional, your emotional mind may feel differently from time to time.

You've learned that it's important to establish healthy boundaries for yourself, find more productive ways to communicate, incorporate good self-care, and be aware of roadblocks to relational satisfaction. But to set yourself free from the emotional ties that bind you to feelings of anger and resentment toward your partner, you need to consider forgiveness.

The issue of forgiveness is a tough one, and it can be hard to let go of the hurts that your partner's ADHD has inflicted on you. But think about it; what is the alternative? What good does it do to hold on to resentments? What will it get you? According to Katherine Piderman, staff chaplain at the Mayo Clinic (quoted in Mayo Clinic 2009), the benefits of forgiveness include greater spiritual and psychological well-being; less personal stress; physical benefits, such as lowered blood pressure and less chronic pain; and from a psychological standpoint, less anxiety and depression, and a lowered risk of alcohol or substance abuse. The freedom that comes from letting go of anger, resentment, and bitterness are best illustrated in the following story.

• Li-Li and Her Mother-in-Law

In Chinese folklore, a long time ago in China, a girl named Li-Li got married and went to live with her husband and mother-in-law. Li-Li found that she couldn't get along at all with her mother-in-law. Their personalities were very different, and many of her mother-in-law's habits made Li-Li angry. In addition, the mother-in-law criticized Li-Li consistently. Li-Li and her mother-in-law constantly argued and fought. But worse, according to ancient Chinese tradition, Li-Li had to submit to her mother-in-law and obey her every wish. All the anger and unhappiness in the house caused Li-Li's husband great distress.

Finally, Li-Li could not stand her mother-in-law's bad temper and dictatorship any longer, so she decided to do something about it. She went to see a man in her village who sold herbs, Mr. Huang. She told him the situation and asked if he would give her some poison so that she could solve the problem once and for all.

Mr. Huang thought for a while and finally said, "Li-Li, I will help you solve your problem, but you must listen to me and obey what I tell you." Li-Li responded, "Yes, Mr. Huang, I will do whatever you tell me to do." Mr. Huang went into the back room and returned in a few minutes with a package of herbs. He told her, "You cannot use a quick-acting poison to get rid of your mother-in-law, because that would cause people to become suspicious. Therefore, I have given you a number of herbs that will slowly build up poison in her body. Every other day, prepare some delicious meal and put a little of these herbs in her serving. Now, to make sure that nobody suspects you when she dies, you must be very careful to act very friendly toward her. Don't argue with her, obey her every wish, and treat her like a queen." Li-Li was so happy. She thanked Mr. Huang and hurried home to put her plan into action.

Weeks and months went by, and every other day, Li-Li served the specially treated food to her mother-in-law. She remembered what Mr. Huang had said about avoiding suspicion, so she controlled her temper, obeyed her mother-in-law, and treated her like her own mother. After six months had passed, the whole household had changed. Li-Li had practiced controlling her temper so much that she found that she almost never got mad or upset. She hadn't had an argument with her mother-in-law in six months because she now seemed much kinder and easier to get along with. The mother-in-law's attitude toward Li-Li had changed too, and she began to treat Li-Li like her own daughter. She kept telling friends and relatives that Li-Li was the best daughter-in-law one could ever find. They were now treating each other in a very loving manner. Li-Li's husband was very happy to see what was happening.

One day, Li-Li went to see Mr. Huang to ask for his help again. She said, "Mr. Huang, please help me to keep the poison from killing my mother-in-law! She has changed into such a nice woman, and I love her like my own mother. I do not want her to die because of the poison I gave her." Mr. Huang smiled and nodded his head: "Li-Li, there's nothing to worry about. I never gave you any poison. The herbs I gave you were vitamins to improve her health. The only poison was in your mind and your attitude toward her, but that has been all washed away by the love you gave to her."

The story is a clear example of how letting go of negative attitudes can help us to feel differently. It's easier to rid ourselves of negative emotions when we understand that ADHD is a neurobiological disorder and that the behaviors attached to the symptoms that hurt your feelings are usually not intentional. It also helps to keep in mind that your partner really does not like having ADHD; in fact he would do pretty much anything not have it. Give your best effort to refocusing on those attributes that are good and positive about your partner. Also spend time trying to rediscover and remember why you were originally drawn to this relationship. Lara Honos-Webb's book *The Gift of Adult ADD: How to Transform Your Challenges and Build on Your Strengths* (2008) does a good job of reminding us that people with ADHD have unrelenting curiosity that can lead to success, that they have innate leadership capabilities because of their tendency to think outside the box, and that they care deeply and intensely. Your original feelings may be buried under years of inattention, restlessness, distractibility, and impulsivity, but it is worth digging down and discovering again what was there in the first place.

EXERCISE 11.5 FORGIVING YOUR PARTNER

How you structure your forgiveness exercise is a completely personal issue. Some people like to write their thoughts in a letter and give or read it to their partners. Others prefer to say their thoughts out loud, almost as a confession. And others choose to never say anything at all, preferring to keep their thoughts of forgiveness a private journey. How you do it is far less important than deciding to forgive and let go of all the things you have been holding on to. Forgiveness is an act of your will; it does not depend on a feeling or an emotion. I encourage you to think about you, your partner, and your relationship, and find a place in your heart to forgive.

Final Thoughts

Your partner who has ADHD may be completely on board with the diagnosis or very resistant to the idea that there is anything wrong. Regardless of your partner's attitude about ADHD, we have discussed some important steps that can help you feel better about how you choose to live your life.

It is essential that you become proactive in your understanding of ADHD. Continue to educate yourself about the disorder so that you will know what to expect. Reading books and searching the Internet for information will help increase your understanding of ADHD. See if there are any support groups in your area; if not, think about starting one. It is reassuring to know that you are not alone and that other people have similar reactions and experience the same feelings that you do.

By recognizing how your partner's ADHD affects every aspect of your life and the impact it has on your relational and family lives, you will be able to manage your own reactions in the healthiest way possible. Use the skills suggested in this book to raise your self-awareness. Use your new self-awareness to develop healthy personal boundaries. Always be conscious of ways to improve your communication skills, and seek out positive ways to resolve conflictual situations. Don't leave your partner who has ADHD out of the process; think of ways to engage him in a manner that is positive and encouraging. Find goals to work toward together.

I can't overemphasize the importance of finding competent clinicians. A therapist who understands all of the components of ADHD and can help you and your partner navigate the choppy waters of an ADHD relationship can be invaluable. Just as important is finding a physician—preferably one who specializes in the medical management of neurobiological disorders—who will work with you and your partner to determine appropriate treatment for ADHD. Ideally, your therapist and your doctor will work together for the best possible outcome.

Continue to find ways to be supportive, understanding, and compassionate. Keep your sense of humor and remember, it's never too late to make changes. Don't give up on your partner who has ADHD, and don't give up on yourself.

Resources

ADDvance (Answers to Your Questions about ADD [ADHD])	addvance.com
Attention Deficit Disorder Association (ADDA)	www.add.org
Attention Deficit Disorder Resources	addresources.org
Children and Adults with Attention Deficit/ Hyperactivity Disorder (CHADD)	chadd.org
National Resource Center on ADHD	help4adhd.org

References

Adler, L. A. 2008. "Epidemiology, Impairments, and Differential Diagnosis in Adult ADHD: Introduction." *CNS Spectrums* 13 (8) (Suppl. 12):4–5.

American Psychiatric Association (APA). 2000. *Diagnostic and Statistical Manual of Mental Disorders (DSM-IV-TR)*. 4th ed., text rev. Arlington, VA: American Psychiatric Association.

Antai-Otong, D. 2008. "The Art of Prescribing Pharmacological Management of Adult ADHD: Implications for Psychiatric Care." *Perspectives in Psychiatric Care* 44 (3):196–201.

Betchen, S. J. 2003. "Suggestions for Improving Intimacy in Couples in Which One Partner Has Attention-Deficit/Hyperactivity Disorder." *Journal of Sex and Marital Therapy* 29 (2):103–24.

Biederman, J., and S. V. Faraone. 2005. "Attention-Deficit Hyperactivity Disorder." *Lancet* 366 (9481):237–48.

Dodson, W. W. 2005. "Pharmacotherapy of Adult ADHD." *Journal of Clinical Psychology* 61 (5):589–606.

Feifel, D., and K. MacDonald. 2008. "Attention-Deficit/Hyperactivity Disorder in Adults: Recognition and Diagnosis of This Often-Overlooked Condition." *Postgraduate Medicine* 120 (3):39–47.

Gilman, L. 2005. "Career Advice from Powerful ADHD and LD Executives: Career Advice from 5 Top Executives Who Transformed Their Attention Deficit Disorder or Learning Disability into an Asset in the Workplace." *ADDitude: Living Well with Attention Deficit*, December/January.

Harvard Health Publications. 2011. "Generalized Anxiety Disorder." *Harvard Mental Health Letter* 27 (12):1–3.

Honos-Webb, L. 2008. *The Gift of Adult ADD: How to Transform Your Challenges and Build on Your Strengths*. Oakland, CA: New Harbinger Publications.

Hughes, R. 2011. "Research Briefs: Artificial Food Dyes and ADHD." *Attention*, June:12–13.

Kessler, R. C., L. Adler, M. Ames, O. Demler, S. Faraone, E. Hiripi, M. J. Howes, R. Jin, K. Secnik, T. Spencer, T. B. Ustun, and E. E. Walters. 2005. "The World Health Organization Adult ADHD Self-Report Scale (ASRS): A Short Screening Scale for Use in the General Population." *Psychological Medicine* 35 (2):245–56.

Kessler, R. C., L. Adler, R. Barkley, J. Biederman, C. K. Conners, O. Demler, S. V. Faraone, L. L. Greenhill, M. J. Howes, K. Secnik, T. Spencer, T. B. Ustun, E. E. Walters, and A. M. Zaslavsky. 2006. "The Prevalence and Correlates of Adult ADHD in the United States: Results from the National Comorbidity Survey Replication." *American Journal of Psychiatry* 163 (4):716–23.

Mayo Clinic. 2009. "Forgiveness: Letting Go of Grudges and Bitterness." Mayo Foundation for Medical Education and Research (MFMER), November 21.

Laaser, M. 1999. *Talking to Your Kids about Sex: How to Have a Lifetime of Age-Appropriate Conversations with Your Children about Healthy Sexuality*. Colorado Springs, CO: WaterBrook Press.

Milich, R., A. C. Balentine, and D. R. Lynam. 2001. "ADHD Combined Type and ADHD Predominantly Inattentive Type Are Distinct and Unrelated Disorders." *Clinical Psychology: Science and Practice* 8 (4):463–88.

Newcorn, J. H. 2008. "Comorbidity in Adults with ADHD." *Primary Psychiatry* 15:8 (Suppl. 4):12–15.

Painter, C. A., F. Prevatt, and T. Welles. 2008. "Career Beliefs and Job Satisfaction in Adults with Symptoms of Attention-Deficit/ Hyperactivity Disorder." *Journal of Employment Counseling* 45 (4):178–87.

Pew Forum on Religion and Public Life. 2010. "Pew Forum on Religion and Public Life Religious Knowledge Survey, May 2010." Pew Forum on Religion and Public Life Poll Database, Washington, DC.

Ramsay, J. R. 2002. "A Cognitive Therapy Approach for Treating Chronic Procrastination and Avoidance: Behavioral Activation Interventions." *Journal of Group Psychotherapy, Psychodrama, and Sociometry* 55:79–92.

Resnick, R. J. 2005. "Attention Deficit Hyperactive Disorder in Teens and Adults: They Don't All Outgrow It." *Journal of Clinical Psychology* 61 (5):529–33.

Richardson, W. 1997. *The Link between A.D.D. and Addiction: Getting the Help You Deserve.* Colorado Springs, CO: Piñon Press.

Smith, B. H., B. S. G. Molina, and W. E. Pelham. 2002. "The Clinically Meaningful Link between Alcohol Use and Attention Deficit Hyperactivity Disorder." *Alcohol Research and Health* 26 (2):122–29.

Spencer, T. J. 2008. "Question-and-Answer Session." *CNS Spectrums* 13 (8) (Suppl. 12):16 –17.

Stein, M. A. 2008. "Impairment Associated with Adult ADHD." *CNS Spectrums* 13 (8) (Suppl. 12):9–11.

Stevens, T., and M. Mulsow. 2006. "There is No Meaningful Relationship between Television Exposure and Symptoms of Attention-Deficit/Hyperactivity Disorder." *Pediatrics* 117 (3):665–72.

Toner, M., T. O'Donoghue, and S. Houghton. 2006. "Living in Chaos and Striving for Control: How Adults with Attention Deficit

Hyperactivity Disorder Deal with Their Disorder." *International Journal of Disability, Development, and Education* 53 (2):247–61.

Wadsworth, J. S., and D. C. Harper. 2007. "Adults with Attention-Deficit/Hyperactivity Disorder: Assessment and Treatment Strategies." *Journal of Counseling and Development* 85 (1):101–109.

Worcester, S. 2010. "Study: Evidence of Genetic Basis for ADHD." *Pediatric News*, October, 6–7.

Zimmerman, F. J., and D. A. Christakis. 2007. "Associations between Content Types of Early Media Exposure and Subsequent Attentional Problems." *Pediatrics* 120 (5):986–92.

Susan Tschudi, MA, is a licensed marriage and family therapist in private practice in Westlake Village, CA, and adjunct professor of psychology at Pepperdine University. As a relationship expert, she specializes in helping couples achieve marital success. She also speaks both nationally and internationally on the subject of attention deficit disorder and relationships. Visit www.lovingsomeonewithadd.com for more information.

MORE BOOKS *from*
NEW HARBINGER PUBLICATIONS

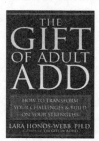
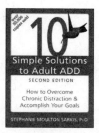
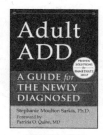
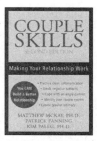
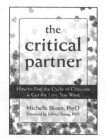
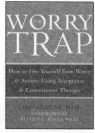